Placenta Accreta Syndrome

Series in Maternal-Fetal Medicine

Operative Obstetrics
Joseph Apuzzio, Anthony M. Vintzileos, Vincenzo Berghella MD, Jesus R. Alvarez-Perez

**The Long-Term Impact of Medical Complications in Pregnancy:
A Window into Maternal and Fetal Future Health**
Eyal Sheiner

Textbook of Diabetes and Pregnancy, Third Edition
Moshe Hod, Lois G. Jovanovic, Gian Carlo Di Renzo, Alberto De Leiva, Oded Langer

Recurrent Pregnancy Loss: Causes, Controversies, and Treatment, Second Edition
Howard J. A. Carp

Neurology and Pregnancy: Clinical Management
Michael S. Marsh, Lina Nashef, Peter Brex

**Fetal Cardiology: Embryology, Genetics, Physiology, Echocardiographic Evaluation,
Diagnosis and Perinatal Management of Cardiac Diseases**
Simcha Yagel, Norman H. Silverman, Ulrich Gembruch

Placenta Accreta Syndrome

Edited by

Robert M. Silver, M.D.

Co-Director of Labor and Delivery
Chief, Division of Maternal–Fetal Medicine
Interim Chair, Department of Obstetrics/Gynecology
University of Utah Health Sciences Center
Salt Lake City, Utah

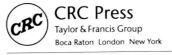

CRC Press
Taylor & Francis Group
Boca Raton London New York

CRC Press is an imprint of the
Taylor & Francis Group, an **informa** business

CRC Press
Taylor & Francis Group
6000 Broken Sound Parkway NW, Suite 300
Boca Raton, FL 33487-2742

© 2017 by Taylor & Francis Group, LLC
CRC Press is an imprint of Taylor & Francis Group, an Informa business

No claim to original U.S. Government works

Printed on acid-free paper

International Standard Book Number-13: 978-1-4987-4596-3 (Paperback)

Library of Congress Cataloging-in-Publication Data

Names: Silver, Robert M., editor.
Title: Placenta accreta syndrome / [edited by] Robert M. Silver.
Other titles: Series in maternal-fetal medicine ; 7. 2158-0855
Description: Boca Raton, FL : CRC Press, Taylor & Francis Group, [2017] | Series: Series in maternal-fetal medicine ; 7 | Includes bibliographical references and index.
Identifiers: LCCN 2016044635| ISBN 9781498745963 (pbk. : alk. paper) | ISBN 9781498746007 (ebook) | ISBN 9781498745970 (ebook)
Subjects: | MESH: Placenta Accreta
Classification: LCC RG591 | NLM WQ 212 | DDC 618.3/4--dc23
LC record available at https://lccn.loc.gov/2016044635

Visit the Taylor & Francis Web site at
http://www.taylorandfrancis.com

and the CRC Press Web site at
http://www.crcpress.com

Contents

Preface

Placenta accreta or morbidly adherent placenta (MAP) is one of the most dangerous conditions encountered in pregnancy. It is associated with considerable maternal morbidity including large volume blood transfusion, need for hysterectomy, intensive care unit (ICU) admission, infection, and prolonged hospitalization. Hemorrhage may be fatal or can lead to disseminated intravascular coagulation (DIC) and multiorgan failure. In fact, the average blood loss at the time of delivery for women with placenta accreta has been reported to be 3000–5000 mL. Other maternal risks include surgical injuries to pelvic viscera and fistula formation. Fetal risks are also considerable and for the most part are due to complications of preterm birth.

Rates of placenta accreta are dramatically increasing, primarily due to the increase in the rate of cesarean delivery. The incidence in the United States has increased from a reported 1 in 30,000 in the 1960s to 1 in 500–700 in the last decade. The overwhelming risk factor for placenta accreta is multiple prior cesarean deliveries. The vast majority of women with accreta have had at least one prior cesarean delivery, and the risk increases with the number of cesarean deliveries. The combination of placenta previa and prior cesarean dramatically increases the risk since the placenta overlies the uterine scar. Indeed, women with two or more prior cesareans and a placenta previa are at extreme risk for placenta accreta. Since the rate of cesarean deliveries continues to escalate, the rate of placenta accreta is expected to increase as well.

Despite increasing frequency of the condition, many aspects of the pathophysiology of placenta accreta as well as the optimal method of diagnosis and management of the condition are uncertain. Each center cares for only a relatively small number of cases per year, making formal study of the condition difficult. Consequently, there are no randomized clinical trials and few prospective studies of any design focusing on this increasingly common, life-threatening condition. For example, many believe that cesarean hysterectomy is the safest way to manage accreta based on limited data that shows improved outcomes compared to expectant management leaving the uterus in place. Others advocate conservative management leaving the placenta in situ and awaiting spontaneous involution. There are dozens of such controversies and uncertainties.

We hope that this book will help clinicians caring for these critically ill women. All aspects of diagnosis and treatment of suspected MAP are addressed and controversies are highlighted. Chapters address a diverse array of topics including epidemiology, pathophysiology, diagnosis with ultrasound and magnetic resource imaging (MRI), and all aspects of management. We are fortunate to have an impressive group of authors with multidisciplinary expertise, including anesthesia, maternal–fetal medicine, gynecologic surgery and oncology, radiology, and hematology. Indeed, they are some of the most experienced MAP clinicians in the world. We are indebted to these terrific authors for sharing their experience and expertise.

Robert M. Silver

Contributors

Alfred Abuhamad
Department of Obstetrics and Gynecology
Eastern Virginia Medical School
Norfolk, Virginia

Thomas Archer
Department of Anesthesiology
University of California
San Diego, California

Eliza M. Berkley
Department of Obstetrics and Gynecology
Eastern Virginia Medical School
Norfolk, Virginia

Michael A. Belfort
Department of Obstetrics and Gynecology
Department of Surgery
Department of Anesthesiology
Baylor College of Medicine
Houston, Texas
and
Division of Maternal Fetal Medicine
Department of Obstetrics and Gynecology
Texas Children's Hospital
Houston, Texas

Amar Bhide
Fetal Medicine Unit
Department of Obstetrics and Gynaecology
St. George's Hospital
London, United Kingdom

Michele A. Brown
Department of Radiology
University of California San Diego School
    of Medicine
La Jolla, California

William M. Burke
Columbia University College of Physicians
    and Surgeons
New York, New York

Graham J. Burton
The Centre for Trophoblast Research
Department of Physiology, Development,
    and Neuroscience
University of Cambridge
Cambridge, United Kingdom

Daniela Carusi
Brigham & Women's Hospital
Harvard Medical School
Boston, Massachusetts

Carolyn Haunschild
Department of Obstetrics and Gynecology
Stanford University School of Medicine
Stanford, California

Karin A. Fox
Department of Obstetrics and Gynecology
Maternal Fetal Medicine Fellowship Program
Maternal Fetal Surgery Section
Baylor College of Medicine
Houston, Texas
and
Division of Maternal Fetal Medicine
Department of Obstetrics and Gynecology
Texas Children's Hospital Pavilion for Women
Houston, Texas

Andrew D. Hull
Department of Reproductive Medicine
University of California San Diego School
    of Medicine
La Jolla, California

Andra H. James
Department of Obstetrics and Gynecology
Duke University
Durham, North Carolina

Eric Jauniaux
UCL Institute for Women's Health
University College London
London, United Kingdom

Gilles Kayem
Department of Obstetrics and Gynecology
Trousseau Hospital, AP-HP
Paris, France

Evelyn Lockhart
Department of Pathology
University of New Mexico
Albuquerque, New Mexico

Deirdre Lyell
Department of Obstetrics and Gynecology
Stanford University School of Medicine
Stanford, California

Erin Martin
Department of Anesthesiology
University of California
San Diego, California

Michael P. Nageotte
Maternal-Fetal Medicine
Miller's Women's & Children's Hospital
Long Beach Memorial Medical Center
Long Beach, California

Annette Perez-Delboy
Columbia University College of Physicians
   and Surgeons
New York, New York

Gladys A. Ramos
Division of Perinatology
Department of Reproductive Medicine
University of California San Diego Health System
San Diego, California

Loïc Sentilhes
Department of Obstetrics and Gynecology
Bordeaux University Hospital
Bordeaux, France

Alireza A. Shamshirsaz
Department of Maternal Fetal Medicine
Baylor College of Medicine
Houston, Texas
and
Division of Maternal Fetal Medicine
Department of Obstetrics and Gynecology
Texas Children's Hospital Pavilion for Women
Houston, Texas

Vineet K. Shrivastava
Maternal-Fetal Medicine
Miller's Women's & Children's Hospital
Long Beach Memorial Medical Center
Long Beach, California

Robert M. Silver
Department of Obstetrics and Gynecology
University of Utah School of Medicine
Salt Lake City, Utah

Jason D. Wright
Columbia University College of Physicians
   and Surgeons
New York, New York

1

Placenta Accreta: Epidemiology and Risk Factors

Daniela Carusi

CONTENTS

Placenta accreta represents one of the most morbid conditions in modern obstetrics, with high rates of hemorrhage, hysterectomy, and intensive care unit admission.[1] By most accounts, placenta accreta appears to be on the rise,[2–4] paralleling the rise in cesarean section rate as a major risk factor. In fact, the true incidence of placenta accreta is difficult to determine, owing to marked variation in the definition of accreta and heterogeneity in the populations studied. This chapter interprets available data on incidence, mortality, and risk factors for placenta accreta.

Definition

Placenta accreta is strictly defined as direct attachment of the placental trophoblast to the uterine myometrium, with no normal intervening decidua or basalis layer.[5] Cases with partial or complete invasion of trophoblast through the uterine wall are called increta and percreta, respectively, though all three categories are collectively identified as "accreta" in the epidemiologic literature. The definition has been further categorized based on the amount of placenta involved, with a "total" accreta involving the entire placenta, while "partial" or "focal" accretas involve individual cotyledons or areas within a cotyledon, respectively.[6]

    The first published review of accreta focused on clinical rather than pathologic diagnosis, specifying "undue adherence of the placenta" to the uterine wall.[5] More recently, the term "morbidly adherent placenta" has been used to define accreta clinically, though exact diagnostic criteria still vary from study to study. Most researchers using a clinical definition identify "difficult," or "piecemeal" removal of the placenta,[7–10] sometimes specifying an antecedent prolonged third stage of labor following a vaginal delivery.[11] Some also specify placental bed hemorrhage after a difficult removal,[3,8,9] though not all authors require a morbidity factor in the diagnosis. Others have allowed a very broad clinical definition, including any postpartum curettage for retained products of conception.[7]

1

Concerns over diagnostic specificity have led some authors to require histologic confirmation, excluding cases that were suspected clinically but lacked pathologic evidence.[12,13] However, reliable pathologic results may not be available when the uterus is conserved, or when multicenter or national-level data are collected.[14–16] Some have conversely emphasized a clinical definition, arguing that adherence and morbidity are the most relevant features of accreta.[6] In fact, some studies have shown that microscopic findings of accreta have a clinical correlation only 11%–33% of the time, suggesting that isolated histologic criteria may also be nonspecific.[17,18] To date, no universal, strict definition exists for data collection purposes.

Incidence

Accreta incidence estimates will be influenced both by the definition used and the specific population of patients studied. Table 1.1 details various estimates according to these factors. When using either a clinical or pathologic diagnosis, regardless of previa status or mode of delivery, general incidence ranges from 1/533 to 1/731 deliveries.[9,13,14]

TABLE 1.1

Studies Reporting Accreta Incidence

Study and Years Investigated	Accreta Incidence	Patient Source	Definition	Notes
Hospital-Level Data Collection				
Clark et al.[19]: 1977–1983	*All deliveries: 1/3372* Previas only: 1/10	Single teaching hospital, United States	Not given	Accreta diagnosed only with previa
Miller et al.[12]: 1985–1994	*All deliveries: 1/2510* Previas only: 1/11 Prior CS only: 1/396	Single teaching hospital, United States	All *histologically* confirmed	Accretas diagnosed either with previa or with hysterectomy
Zaki et al.[20]: 1990–1996	*All deliveries: 1/1922* Previas only: 1/9	Single hospital, Saudi Arabia	*Clinical*	Accreta diagnosed only with previa
Gielchinsky et al.[7]: 1990–2000	*All deliveries: 1/111* Previas only: 1/10	Single hospital, Israel	*Clinical* or *histologic*	Used broad clinical criteria, including ultrasound findings of RPOC requiring curettage
Wu et al.[9]: 1982–2002	*All deliveries: 1/533*	Single teaching hospital, United States	*Clinical* or *histologic*	Excluded women with fbroids; gravida 1 patients excluded from risk factor analysis
Silver et al.[10]: 1999–2002	Unlabored CS only: 1/211 Primary unlabored CS only: 1/333	19 academic centers, United States	*Clinical* or *histologic*	Evaluated unlabored CSs only
Usta et al.[8]: 1983–2003	Previas only: 1/16	Single teaching hospital, Lebanon	*Clinical* or *histologic*	Included cases of previa only
Morlando et al.[3]: 1976–2008	*All deliveries: 1976–1978: 1/833 2006–2008: 1/322*	Single teaching hospital, Italy	*Clinical* or *histologic*	Rising CS rate over time period: 17%–64%
Esh-Broder et al.[13]: 2004–2009	*All deliveries: 1/599*	Single teaching hospital, Israel	*Clinical* and *histologic*	Searched all pathology reports
Eshkoli et al.[21]: 1988–2011	Singleton CS only: 1/250	Single tertiary center, Israel	*Clinical*	Included singleton cesarean deliveries only
Bailit et al.[14]: 2008–2011	*All deliveries: 1/731*	25 hospitals (22/25 teaching hospitals), United States	*Clinical*	Evaluated a random sample of deliveries during the time period

(Continued)

TABLE 1.1 *(Continued)*

Studies Reporting Accreta Incidence

Study and Years Investigated	Accreta Incidence	Patient Source	Definition	Notes
National-Level Data Collection				
Upson et al.[16]: 2005–2010	*All deliveries: 1/1136 2005: 1/1266 2010: 1/943*	National discharge data, Ireland	Discharge coding	ICD-10 codes for MAP and some form of accreta
Mehrabadi et al.[22]: 2009–2010	*All deliveries: 1/694*	National coding, Canadian Institute for Health Information	Canadian Health System ICD coding	Used unique codes for accreta
Fitzpatrick et al.[23]: 2010–2011	*All deliveries: 1/5882 No prior CS: 1/33,000 Previa and prior CS: 1/20*	National, centralized data collection, United Kingdom	*Clinical or histologic*	Cases tracked by clinicians, mailed in to central unit for review
Thurn et al.[15]: 2009–2012	*All deliveries: 1/2953 Broad definition: 1/2162*	International database: collaboration of Nordic countries	Mailed in surveys plus search of ICD-10 coding *Clinical only*	If vaginal delivery, must go to laparotomy and have transfusion to be included; "broad definition" included those diagnosed as not having laparotomy after vaginal delivery

Abbreviations: CS, cesarean section; ICD, International Classification of Diseases; MAP, morbidly adherent placenta; RPOC, retained products of conception.

Table 1.1 lists studies that report accreta incidence, specifying the population studied and definitions used. Higher estimates are obtained when a broad clinical definition is used (1/111 with the inclusion of retained products of conception)[7] or when the analysis is restricted to higher risk patients. An incidence of 1/211 deliveries was obtained when evaluating only patients undergoing an unlabored cesarean section (which will preferentially select those with previa), with a slightly lower rate of 1/333 obtained after excluding repeat cesarean sections.[10] An additional study evaluating only cesarean deliveries found a similar rate of 1/250.[21]

Relatively lower incidences are reported when using stricter definitions of accreta. Early studies diagnosed an accreta only in the setting of placenta previa, and found rates of 1/1922 to 1/2510.[12,20] Thus, it is difficult to confirm a rising incidence of accreta over time, as the increase may reflect differences in definitions and patient populations. Few centers have reported time trends internally. One center in Southern Italy showed a linear rise in accreta incidence over four decades, from 1/833 to 1/322 deliveries. Of note, its cesarean section rate correspondingly rose from 16% to over 60%, supporting the role of this factor in the observed increase.[3] Another study tracking national discharge data found a rate of 1/1266 in 2005 that increased to 1/943 in 2010.

It is important to note that the majority of these studies report accreta incidence within academic or tertiary medical centers, which likely care for a disproportionately large number of accreta patients, some of whom may be referred for care. Accordingly, hospital rates may not reflect population rates. For example, Bailit et al. reported an incidence of 1/731 using a large sample of US deliveries, though 22 of the 25 included hospitals were academic centers.[14] In this context, rising incidence rates may not reflect a true increase in accreta occurrence, but rather improved antepartum diagnosis and referral patterns. Unfortunately, it is not possible to calculate the actual incidence of placenta accreta across the United States, as the condition is not accurately captured with available discharge diagnosis coding. While the ninth edition of the International Classification of Diseases (ICD-9 CM) contains no code for placenta accreta, this diagnosis was included and introduced nationwide in 2015 in the tenth edition of ICD-10 CM.[24] This should allow better future estimates of nationwide incidence, albeit in the absence of strict diagnostic criteria.

Other developed countries have been able to estimate their national accreta incidences, and as expected, the numbers are lower than those reported in tertiary centers. Fitzpatrick et al. performed a 1-year study in the United Kingdom from 2010 to 2011, in which all delivering providers were asked to prospectively report accreta cases to a central registry. After confirming the diagnoses, they reported an overall incidence of 1/5882 deliveries.[23] Ireland began using ICD-10 coding in 2005, allowing calculation of its 5-year accreta incidence at 1/1136 using discharge codes.[16] Capturing 91% of deliveries, an international collaboration of Nordic countries reported an accreta incidence of 1/2162, based on provider reporting and discharge coding, though inconsistently requiring both.[15] Finally, Canada, with the exclusion of Quebec, was found to have a 1/692 incidence of accreta using a national discharge coding system.[22] The wide range in these reported national statistics may reflect the lack of standard diagnostic criteria, and perhaps variation in risk factors such as cesarean rates, parity, and cesarean technique.

Mortality

While uncommon, placenta accreta contributes substantially to major maternal morbidity.[1] A maternal mortality rate of 7% has been quoted by a number of reviews, which is alarmingly high.[2,4,25] This number originated from a survey of maternal–fetal medicine specialists, which focused on placenta percreta, and obtained a 23% response rate.[26] While 7% of cases reported in the survey and at the author's home institution resulted in a maternal death, this number is likely inflated by reporting bias. Furthermore, placenta percreta is the most morbid and least common of accreta variants.

Without knowing the total number of accreta cases in the United States, the national accreta mortality rate cannot be precisely calculated. However, the rate for individual populations can be known when complete series of accreta cases are published. Reviewing such series, a single medical center in Saudi Arabia reported one death out of 12 previa accretas (8%) treated between 1990 and 1996.[20] In contrast, two separate series from the University of Southern California reported no maternal deaths out of 91 total previa accretas, which is significantly lower than the 7% rate previously reported.[12,19] Using a much more liberal definition of accreta, which would be expected to decrease the mortality rate by increasing the denominator, an Israeli center reported one death among 310 accretas (0.3%).[7] More recently, the Nordic collaborative study reported no maternal deaths among 205 accretas,[15] while the Canadian national study identified one death among 819 accreta cases (0.12%).[22] Multiple other published series made no mention of maternal deaths, including a total of 321 cases diagnosed at mainly tertiary or academic centers,[9,13,14] and 357 cases identified in Ireland using discharge data. This may reflect a disproportionately low mortality rate in experienced centers, or likely reporting bias.

These case series suggest that the actual case-fatality rate from placenta accreta is lower than the oft-quoted 7%, though the true rate will likely vary based on type of accreta, patient comorbidities, and the delivery location. Given that accreta stands out as one of the most morbid maternal conditions in modern obstetrics, careful patient counseling and appropriate referral remain critical.

Risk Factors

Table 1.2 lists reported risk factors for placenta accreta, categorized by strength and consistency of evidence. Placenta previa and history of a prior cesarean delivery comprise the strongest, most-cited risk factors for placenta accreta. Pathophysiologically, accreta is believed to result from trophoblast attachment to a deficient or damaged area of uterine decidua.[2] Insufficient endometrium in the area of the lower uterine segment and damage at the area of a prior cesarean section scar may facilitate this process. Other risk factors have been less consistently established, perhaps due to the dominance of these two factors, as well as variations in individual study design.

Notably, the first published series of 18 clinical and pathologic accretas included only one patient with placenta previa and one with prior cesarean section. These authors highlighted prior events that

TABLE 1.2

Risk Factors for Placenta Accreta

Consistent Evidence from Controlled Studies
• Placenta previa • Prior CS(s) (particularly with a placenta previa) • In vitro fertilization (IVF)
Inconsistent evidence from controlled studies
• Maternal age ≥35 • Prior dilation and curettage of the uterus • Prior myomectomy or other uterine surgery (besides CS) • Maternal smoking
Anecdotal evidence from case series and reports
• Prior history of accreta • Uterine synechiae or Asherman's syndrome • Prior endometrial ablation • Prior uterine fibroid embolization • Congenital uterine anomalies (such as a rudimentary horn) • Prior uterine irradiation

Abbreviations: CS, cesarean section; IVF, in vitro fertilization.

may have damaged the endometrium, including manual extraction of the placenta, uterine sepsis, and curettage as potential risk factors.[5] As US cesarean section rates have risen dramatically—from 4.5% to 32.7% over the past half-century[27,28]—the typical case of accreta has transformed as well.

Placenta Previa

Previa is the dominant modern risk factor for placenta accreta, with reported odds ratios greater than 50.[11,15,23] Accreta incidences of 1/9 to 1/16 have been observed among patients with placenta previa at the time of delivery (Table 1.1).[7,8,12,20] Correspondingly, some researchers have studied the condition only in the context of a previa, allowing easier identification of accreta patients, but precluding identification of other independent risk factors.[12,19,20] Similarly, the majority of studies on antenatal accreta diagnosis have focused on patients with placenta previa, or low anterior placental implantations.[29] Current research is needed on the identification, morbidity, and management of accretas occurring without placenta previa.

Prior Cesarean Section

A history of one or multiple cesareans has been linked to accreta risk, with some showing a linear increase in both previa and accreta risk based on the number of prior cesarean sections.[8,9,12,15,19,30,31] The risk is higher when the placenta is implanted over the prior cesarean scar (as opposed to a posterior placenta previa).[8,12] A 2005 study found that prior cesarean was not a significant independent predictor of accreta, but this study had limited power to show the association (the odds ratio was 2.3 for prior cesarean section, with a confidence interval that crossed one).[11] In contrast, a larger, multinational study showed that prior cesarean was associated with accreta after controlling for other risk factors, including previa.[15] As previously mentioned, the rising rate of cesarean section is often implicated in the rising observed accreta incidence.[2,4,25]

Details of the prior cesarean may impact the subsequent risk for accreta. For example, accreta was found to be more likely when the prior hysterotomy was closed with continuous rather than interrupted sutures[32] or when the prior cesarean was elective (unlabored) versus emergent.[33] Another study found shorter cesarean-to-conception time intervals with placenta accreta than with non-accreta controls.[34] This relationship was not found in accretas following a prior vaginal birth.[34] Given the large number of factors that may differ with cesarean section, cause-and-effect hypotheses need to be confirmed with larger controlled human studies and animal models. Nevertheless, the potential to reduce later risk with surgical technique is encouraging.

Accreta risk factors beyond previa and prior cesarean section have been demonstrated less consistently. Using a large, multicenter cohort of women undergoing cesarean deliveries, Bowman et al. found no additional independent risk factors beyond placenta previa and number of prior cesareans when using a multivariable analysis.[35] In contrast, Thurn et al.[15] found that 31% of patients with an adherent placenta had neither a previa or a prior cesarean section, and others have identified additional independent risk factors. To date the pathophysiology and clinical behavior of accreta outside of the context of placenta previa is less well defined.

Maternal Age

Advanced maternal age, defined as 35 years old or greater, is commonly implicated in accreta risk. While it may be a marker for higher parity and placenta previa risk,[36] some have found it to be an independent accreta risk factor.[9,11,16,21] Others found no association with age when limiting analysis to previa and controlling for prior cesarean section,[8] while another found that age was relevant only among women who had not undergone a prior cesarean section.[23] These studies vary in terms of case ascertainment and choice of covariates for their models, which may explain the disparate results.

Other Uterine Surgery

Using a national UK database, Fitzpatrick et al. noted that surgery other than prior cesarean was associated with accreta, with a significant odds ratio of 3.4. This included a range of prior procedures, including myomectomy, uterine curettage, and termination of pregnancy. It also included manual extraction of a placenta and removal of retained products of conception, which could be markers for prior placenta accreta.[23] Others found no independent association, using a broad category of "uterine surgery."[11,16] A 2012 study reported no association between accreta and prior myomectomy, though it is important to note that they compared women with prior myomectomy to women with prior low transverse cesarean section.[37] This suggests that the accreta risk is comparable with the two types of surgery, but does not address whether myomectomy patients have a higher risk than those with no prior uterine surgery.

Prior uterine curettage has been inconsistently implicated as a risk factor. One study showed a significant trend as the number of curettages increased to three or more.[11] However, others reported univariate associations with multiple prior curettages, which disappeared after controlling for confounding variables.[7,8] Prior curettage was not a significant risk factor in an analysis restricted to placenta previa, suggesting that it may not have a role in this specific clinical scenario.[12] Larger studies are needed evaluating this specific risk factor when placenta accreta is found without a previa.

Past Obstetric History

Besides history of cesarean section, identifiable risk factors in a past pregnancy may help predict placenta accreta. The most obvious is a history of prior placenta accreta or adherent placenta. This variable has received little attention, given that accreta often results in hysterectomy. However, as uterine conservation and accreta without previa is increasingly performed and reported, outcomes in subsequent pregnancies are increasingly described. In 30 women undergoing cesarean section with conservative management of accreta, Eshkoli et al. found that 13.3% had accreta in the next pregnancy.[21] Using a less restrictive accreta definition, Sentilhes et al. reported a 28.6% rate of recurrent accreta with 21 subsequent deliveries.[38] Another group evaluated seven pregnancies that followed a treated cesarean section scar implantation (CSI); two (28%) experienced placenta accreta.[39] While patients may feel some reassurance that a normal outcome is possible following conservative management of accreta, women with a history of adherent placentation or CSI should be carefully prepared for morbid placentation in subsequent pregnancies. This issue is explored in more detail in Chapter 7.

Current Pregnancy Factors

Given the importance of antepartum accreta identification and delivery planning, factors beyond second and third trimester ultrasound findings have been evaluated as potential predictors of accreta. The most specific may be identification of a first trimester implantation within the CS scar (see Figure 1.1). While such a finding often leads to pregnancy termination, those who continue their pregnancies should be considered very high risk for placenta accreta. One series of 10 such patients showed a 100% rate of placenta accreta,[40] while a second reported accretas in three of five ongoing pregnancies (60%).[41]

Placental hormones, including maternal serum alpha-fetoprotein (AFP) and free beta-HCG, have been reported to be at significantly higher levels when placenta accreta is present. This is true when comparing accreta to non-accreta pregnancies in general,[11] when comparing hysterectomies for accreta to cesarean hysterectomies for other indications,[42] or when comparing previa accretas to previas without accreta.[43] Of note, the last two comparisons evaluated AFP levels only. While the use of serum markers to identify accreta patients appears promising, appropriate cutoffs and associated predictive values have not been firmly established.

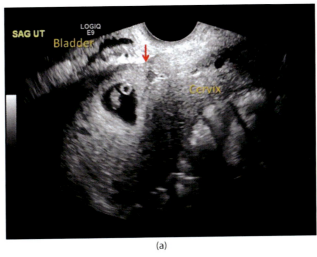

(a)

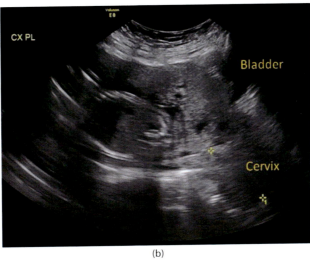

(b)

FIGURE 1.1 Cesarean scar implantation (CSI) evolving into placenta previa/accreta. (a) Ultrasound scan of a 7-week pregnancy implanted at the area of a prior cesarean section scar (red arrow). (b) The same uterus at 20 weeks gestation, now with a complete placenta previa and signs of placenta accreta.

Abnormal Endometrium

Assuming that accreta develops due to abnormalities of the decidual barrier, it is reasonable to link this outcome to abnormally thinned or damaged endometrium. This hypothesis has been supported in a number of different contexts, beyond a history of prior uterine surgery or cesarean section. Pronounced examples of endometrial damage include Asherman's syndrome, involving the endometrium being focally or diffusely replaced by fibrotic scar tissue, and endometrial ablation. While observational data are lacking for these patient groups, case series have described adherent placentas in 2 out of 23 women (9%) who had been treated for Asherman's syndrome[44] and 18/70 women (26%) who had a prior endometrial ablation.[45]

Beyond endometrial damage, endometrial thickness at the time of implantation may play a role as well. Women who undergo in vitro fertilization (IVF) procedures often have direct measures of endometrial thickness prior to conception, and a relatively thinner endometrial lining has been associated with both placenta previa and placenta accreta in women undergoing IVF.[46,47] Cigarette smoking has been associated with thin endometrium in IVF patients,[48] though this association has not been studied in the general population. Smoking has variably been described as a risk factor for placenta accreta, with two studies showing a positive relationship between smoking and accreta,[8,16] while a third showed no association.[21]

The relationship between accreta and additional uterine abnormalities, such as Mullerian anomalies or nonsurgical uterine treatments, has only been described as case reports. Some reports described accretas after prior uterine fibroid embolization, which is often considered a relative contraindication to future pregnancy.[49,50] Accreta has also been noted in two cases of implantation within a rudimentary uterine horn, both resulting in uterine rupture.[51,52] Finally, an unusual case of placenta accreta and early uterine rupture followed prior whole body irradiation.[53]

In Vitro Fertilization

IVF was first reported as a risk factor for accreta in 2011. Since then, multiple studies have shown a significant association, with odds ratios ranging from 2.7 to 32.[13,23,54] This association has held when IVF pregnancies were compared not only to spontaneous conceptions, but also to other fertility treatments, including ovulation induction.[13,54] There are multiple possible explanations for this association, including the role of endometrial receptivity, direct effects on the trophectoderm, or confounding by either maternal history (such as advanced maternal age, prior uterine surgery, or uterine factor infertility) or placenta previa.

Additional studies have shown that cryopreserved embryo transfer (CET) has a higher risk for accreta, retained placenta, and postpartum hemorrhage than a fresh IVF cycle.[55,56] Kaser et al. showed that the association between accreta and CET persisted after controlling for both placenta previa and maternal factors, such as age, prior uterine surgery, uterine factor infertility, and prior cesarean section, suggesting that the role of IVF cannot be explained by confounding alone.[47] This group noted that accreta was associated with a significantly thinner preimplantation endometrium, which occurs in unstimulated CET cycles with uterine preparation. Ovarian stimulation during a fresh IVF cycle produces a significantly thicker endometrial lining, which may be somewhat protective (Figure 1.2). More research in this area is needed to sort out the role of embryo freezing from that of endometrial effects and to determine potential modifiable risk factors for abnormal placentation, such as method of freezing or endometrial preparation.

Notably, the morbidity of placenta accreta in an IVF pregnancy may differ from that of spontaneous pregnancies. Esh-Broder et al. reported no hysterectomies among 12 IVF pregnancies affected by accreta compared to a 13% rate with spontaneous pregnancies, though the rates of previa and prior cesarean section in the two groups were similar.[13] In the Kaser et al. study, 68% of the 50 IVF patients with placenta accreta experienced some type of surgical or hemorrhagic morbidity, though only 8% required a hysterectomy and 30% required a blood transfusion.[47] This may reflect either more focal or less invasive pathology with IVF-related accretas, which is important when counseling patients about the risks of the procedure. Whether this finding extrapolates to non-previa accretas in general needs to be elucidated.

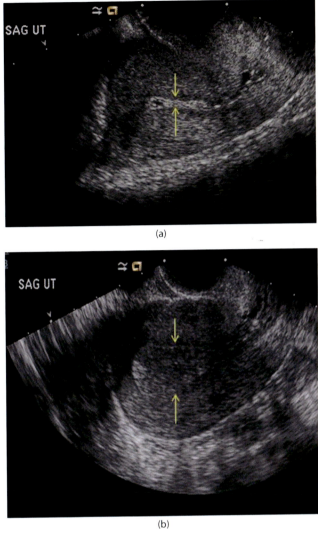

(a)

(b)

FIGURE 1.2 Endometrial thickness measured prior to planned embryo transfer in two in vitro fertilization (IVF) patients. (a) Ultrasound scan shows a very thin endometrium, measuring 2.5 mm (boundaries indicated by arrows). (b) A relatively thick, 16-mm endometrium.

Conclusions

The face of placenta accreta has transformed over the past century. The first large published case series described densely adherent placentas, usually found after vaginal delivery. These women generally had high parity, no placenta previa, and no prior cesarean section.[5] As the cesarean section rate rose substantially during the latter half of the 20th century, placenta accreta was more often described with placenta previa, usually in the setting of one or more prior cesarean sections. While reports in the 1990s described accreta only in the setting of a placenta previa,[12,19,20] later studies again included those without previas and with vaginal deliveries.[9,14]

This reporting trend may correlate with a rise in procedures that impact the endometrium and implantation, including endometrial ablation, hysteroscopic resections, and IVF. As maternal age, assisted reproductive technology, and the use of cryopreserved and donated oocytes rise, we may expect to see more morbidly adherent placentation, both with and without placenta previa. The morbidity related to these deliveries is undeniable, from the first peripartum blood transfusion in 1927 to more recent maternal mortality estimates exceeding one in 1,000 women. Identification of patients at risk and preparation for potentially complicated deliveries will be an important part of reducing this severe morbidity.

Much work remains to understand the incidence and risk factors for placenta accreta. As updated coding systems (ICD-10 CM) allow the capture of national-level discharge data, more accurate estimates of accreta incidence will become available. However, both clinical and pathologic diagnosis at the individual patient level still require standardization. Ultimately, it may make most sense to define accreta as a disease spectrum, distinguishing whether a placenta is merely adherent or truly invasive, the degree of vascularity involved, and whether it is found only histologically or has a clinical correlation. Each of these scenarios may be important in different contexts, such as studying diagnostic tools, anticipating the morbidity of a delivery, understanding accreta's pathophysiology, tracking the disorder's incidence, or counseling patients for future deliveries.

Studies of accreta risk factors are similarly limited. Results will necessarily vary according to the accreta definition used (clinical or pathologic, with previa or without) and the specific set of variables queried. As researchers are able to assemble larger databases, independent risk factors can be elucidated more reliably, though this will also rely on standardized diagnostic criteria. As this work progresses, improvements should be made both in patient identification and management, and ultimately in reducing disease incidence by managing modifiable risk factors.

REFERENCES

1. Grobman WA, Bailit JL, Rice MM et al. Frequency of and factors associated with severe maternal morbidity. *Obstet Gynecol.* 2014 Apr;123(4):804–810. PubMed PMID: 24785608. Pubmed Central PMCID: 4116103.
2. Silver RM. Abnormal placentation: Placenta previa, vasa previa, and placenta accreta. *Obstet Gynecol.* 2015 Sep;126(3):654–668. PubMed PMID: 26244528.
3. Morlando M, Sarno L, Napolitano R et al. Placenta accreta: Incidence and risk factors in an area with a particularly high rate of cesarean section. *Acta Obstet Gynecol Scand.* 2013;92(4):457–460. PubMed PMID: 23347183.
4. Belfort MA. Placenta accreta. *Am J Obstet Gynecol.* 2010 Nov;203(5):430–439. PubMed PMID: 21055510. Epub 2010/11/09.eng.
5. Irving F, Hertig A. A study of placenta accreta. *Surg Gynecol Obstet.* 1937;64:178–200.
6. Fox H. Placenta accreta, 1945–1969. *Obstet Gynecol Surv.* 1972;27(7):475–490.
7. Gielchinsky Y, Rojansky N, Fasouliotis SJ, Ezra Y. Placenta accreta—Summary of 10 years: A survey of 310 cases. *Placenta.* 2002 Feb–Mar; 23(2–3):210–214. PubMed PMID: 11945088.
8. Usta IM, Hobeïka EM, Musa AA, Gabriel GE, Nassar AH. Placenta previa-accreta: Risk factors and complications. *Am J Obstet Gynecol.* 2005;193(3 Pt 2):1045–1049. PubMed PMID: 16157109.
9. Wu S, Kocherginsky M, Hibbard JU. Abnormal placentation: Twenty-year analysis. *Am J Obstet Gynecol.* 2005 May;192(5):1458–1461. PubMed PMID: 15902137.
10. Silver RM, Landon MB, Rouse DJ et al. Maternal morbidity associated with multiple repeat cesarean deliveries. *Obstet Gynecol.* 2006 Jun;107(6):1226–1232. PubMed PMID: 16738145.
11. Hung TH, Shau WY, Hsieh CC, Chiu TH, Hsu JJ, Hsieh TT. Risk factors for placenta accreta. *Obstet Gynecol.* 1999;93(4):545–550.
12. Miller DA, Chollet JA, Goodwin TM. Clinical risk factors for placenta previa-placenta accreta. *Am J Obstet Gynecol.* 1997;177(1):210–214.
13. Esh-Broder E, Ariel I, Abas-Bashir N, Bdolah Y, Celnikier DH. Placenta accreta is associated with IVF pregnancies: A retrospective chart review. *BJOG.* 2011;118(9):1084–1089. PubMed PMID: 21585640.
14. Bailit JL, Grobman WA, Rice MM et al. Morbidly adherent placenta treatments and outcomes. *Obstet Gynecol.* 2015;125(3):683–689. PubMed PMID: 25730233. Pubmed Central PMCID: NIHMS648832 PMC4347990.
15. Thurn L, Lindqvist PG, Jakobsson M et al. Abnormally invasive placenta-prevalence, risk factors and antenatal suspicion: Results from a large population-based pregnancy cohort study in the Nordic countries. *BJOG.* 2015 Jul;123(8):1348–1355. PubMed PMID: 26227006.

16. Upson K, Silver RM, Greene R, Lutomski J, Holt VL. Placenta accreta and maternal morbidity in the Republic of Ireland, 2005–2010. *J Matern Fetal Neonatal Med.* 2014;27(1):24–29. PubMed PMID: 23638753.
17. Jacques SM, Qureshi F, Trent VS, Ramirez NC. Placenta accreta: Mild cases diagnosed by placental examination. *Int J Gynecol Pathol.* 1996;15(1):28–33. PubMed PMID: 8852443.
18. Khong TY, Werger AC. Myometrial fibers in the placental basal plate can confirm but do not necessarily indicate clinical placenta accreta. *Am J Clin Pathol.* 2001 Nov;116(5):703–708. PubMed PMID: 11710687.
19. Clark SL, Koonings PP, Phelan JP. Placenta previa/accreta and prior cesarean section. *Obstet Gynecol.* 1985 Jul;66(1):89–92. PubMed PMID: 4011075.
20. Zaki ZM, Bahar AM, Ali ME, Albar HA, Gerais MA. Risk factors and morbidity in patients with placenta previa accreta compared to placenta previa non-accreta. *Acta Obstet Gynecol Scand.* 1998;77(4):391–394. PubMed PMID: 9598946.
21. Eshkoli T, Weintraub AY, Sergienko R, Sheiner E. Placenta accreta: Risk factors, perinatal outcomes, and consequences for subsequent births. *Am J Obstet Gynecol.* 2013;208(3): 219.e1–e7. PubMed PMID: 23313722.
22. Mehrabadi A, Hutcheon JA, Liu S et al. Contribution of placenta accreta to the incidence of postpartum hemorrhage and severe postpartum hemorrhage. *Obstet Gynecol.* 2015 Apr;125(4):814–821. PubMed PMID: 25751202.
23. Fitzpatrick KE, Sellers S, Spark P, Kurinczuk JJ, Brocklehurst P, Knight M. Incidence and risk factors for placenta accreta/increta/percreta in the UK: A national case-control study. *PloS one.* 2012;7(12):e52893. PubMed PMID: 23300807. Pubmed Central PMCID: 3531337.
24. Centers for Disease Control and Prevention. International Classification of Diseases, tenth Revision, Clinical Modification (ICD-10-CM) 2015. Cited April 7, 2016. Available at: http://www.cdc.gov/nchs/icd/icd10cm.htm.
25. Committee on Obstetric Practice. ACOG committee opinion. Placenta accreta. Number 529, July 2012. American College of Obstetricians and Gynecologists. *Obstet Gynecol.* 2012;120(1):207–211.
26. O'Brien JM, Barton JR, Donaldson ES. The management of placenta percreta: Conservative and operative strategies. *Am J Obstet Gynecol.* 1996 Dec;175(6):1632–1638. PubMed PMID: 8987952.
27. Placek PJ, Taffel S, Moien M. Cesarean section delivery rates: United States, 1981. *Am J Public Health.* 1983 Aug;73(8):861–862. PubMed PMID: 6869638. Pubmed Central PMCID: 1651118.
28. Martin JA, Hamilton BE, Osterman MJ, Curtin SC, Matthews TJ. Births: Final data for 2013. *Natl Vital Stat Rep.* 2015 Jan 15;64(1):1–65. PubMed PMID: 25603115.
29. Comstock CH, Bronsteen RA. The antenatal diagnosis of placenta accreta. *BJOG.* 2014 Jan;121(2):171–181; discussion 181–182. PubMed PMID: 24373591.
30. Daltveit AK, Tollanes MC, Pihlstrom H et al. Cesarean delivery and subsequent pregnancies. *Obstet Gynecol.* 2008 Jun;111(6):1327–1334. PubMed PMID: 18515516.
31. Grobman WA, Gersnoviez R, Landon MB et al. Pregnancy outcomes for women with placenta previa in relation to the number of prior cesarean deliveries. *Obstet Gynecol.* 2007 Dec;110(6):1249–1255. PubMed PMID: 18055717.
32. Sumigama S, Sugiyama C, Kotani T et al. Uterine sutures at prior caesarean section and placenta accreta in subsequent pregnancy: A case-control study. *BJOG.* 2014;121(7):866–874; discussion 75. PubMed PMID: 24666658.
33. Kamara M, Henderson JJ, Doherty DA, Dickinson JE, Pennell CE. The risk of placenta accreta following primary elective caesarean delivery: A case-control study. *BJOG.* 2013 Jun;120(7):879–886. PubMed PMID: 23448347.
34. Wax JR, Seiler A, Horowitz S, Ingardia CJ. Interpregnancy interval as a risk factor for placenta accreta. *Conn Med.* 2000;64(11):659–661.
35. Bowman ZS, Eller AG, Bardsley TR, Greene T, Varner MW, Silver RM. Risk factors for placenta accreta: A large prospective cohort. *Am J Perinatol.* 2014;31(9):799–804. PubMed PMID: 24338130.
36. Gilliam M, Rosenberg D, Davis F. The likelihood of placenta previa with greater number of cesarean deliveries and higher parity. *Obstet Gynecol.* 2002;99(6):976–980. PubMed PMID: 12052584.
37. Gyamfi-Bannerman C, Gilbert S, Landon MB et al. Risk of uterine rupture and placenta accreta with prior uterine surgery outside of the lower segment. *Obstet Gynecol.* 2012 Dec;120(6):1332–1337. PubMed PMID: 23168757. Pubmed Central PMCID: 3545277.

38. Sentilhes L, Kayem G, Ambroselli C et al. Fertility and pregnancy outcomes following conservative treatment for placenta accreta. *Hum Reprod.* 2010 Nov;25(11):2803–2810. PubMed PMID: 20833739.

39. Seow KM, Hwang JL, Tsai YL, Huang LW, Lin YH, Hsieh BC. Subsequent pregnancy outcome after conservative treatment of a previous cesarean scar pregnancy. *Acta Obstet Gynecol Scand.* 2004;83(12):1167–1172. PubMed PMID: 15548150.

40. Timor-Tritsch IE, Monteagudo A, Cali G et al. Cesarean scar pregnancy is a precursor of morbidly adherent placenta. *Ultrasound Obstet Gynecol.* 2014;44(3):346–353. PubMed PMID: 24890256.

41. Michaels AY, Washburn EE, Pocius KD, Benson CB, Doubilet PM, Carusi DA. Outcome of cesarean scar pregnancies diagnosed sonographically in the first trimester. *J Ultrasound Med.* 2015 Apr;34(4): 595–599. PubMed PMID: 25792574.

42. Kupferminc MJ, Tamura RK, Wigton TR, Glassenberg R, Socol ML. Placenta accreta is associated with elevated maternal serum alpha-fetoprotein. *Obstet Gynecol.* 1993;82(2):266–269. PubMed PMID: 7687756.

43. Zelop C, Nadel A, Frigoletto FD Jr, Pauker S, MacMillan M, Benacerraf BR. Placenta accreta/percreta/increta: A cause of elevated maternal serum alpha-fetoprotein. *Obstet Gynecol.* 1992 Oct;80(4): 693–694. PubMed PMID: 1383899.

44. Friedman A, DeFazio J, DeCherney A. Severe obstetric complications after aggressive treatment of Asherman syndrome. *Obstet Gynecol.* 1986;67(6):864–867. PubMed PMID: 3703411.

45. Patni S, ElGarib AM, Majd HS et al. Endometrial resection mandates reliable contraception thereafter—A case report of placenta increta following endometrial ablation. *Eur J Contracept Reprod Health Care.* 2008 Jun;13(2):208–211. PubMed PMID: 18465485.

46. Rombauts L, Motteram C, Berkowitz E, Fernando S. Risk of placenta praevia is linked to endometrial thickness in a retrospective cohort study of 4537 singleton assisted reproduction technology births. *Hum Reprod.* 2014 Dec;29(12):2787–2793. PubMed PMID: 25240011.

47. Kaser DJ, Melamed A, Bormann CL et al. Cryopreserved embryo transfer is an independent risk factor for placenta accreta. *Fertil Steril.* 2015 May;103(5):1176–1184.e2. PubMed PMID: 25747133.

48. Weigert M, Hofstetter G, Kaipl D et al. The effect of smoking on oocyte quality and hormonal parameters of patients undergoing in vitro fertilization-embryo transfer. *J Assist Reprod Genet.* 1999 Jul;16(6): 287–293. PubMed PMID: 10394523. Pubmed Central PMCID: 3455531.

49. El-Miligy M, Gordon A, Houston G. Focal myometrial defect and partial placenta accreta in a pregnancy following bilateral uterine artery embolization. *J Vasc Interv Radiol.* 2007;18(6):789–791. PubMed PMID: 17538144.

50. Takahashi H, Hayashi S, Matsuoka K et al. Placenta accreta following uterine artery embolization. *Taiwan J Obstet Gynecol.* 2010 Jun;49(2):197–198. PubMed PMID: 20708528.

51. Henriet E, Roman H, Zanati J, Lebreton B, Sabourin JC, Loic M. Pregnant noncommunicating rudimentary uterine horn with placenta percreta. *JSLS.* 2008;12(1):101–103. PubMed PMID: 18402750. Pubmed Central PMCID: PMC3016034.

52. Oral B, Guney M, Ozsoy M, Sonal S. Placenta accreta associated with a ruptured pregnant rudimentary uterine horn. Case report and review of the literature. *Arch Gynecol Obstet.* 2001;265(2):100–102.

53. Norwitz ER, Stern HM, Grier H, Lee-Parritz A. Placenta percreta and uterine rupture associated with prior whole body radiation therapy. *Obstet Gynecol.* 2001 Nov;98(5 Pt 2):929–931. PubMed PMID: 11704208.

54. Hayashi M, Nakai A, Satoh S, Matsuda Y. Adverse obstetric and perinatal outcomes of singleton pregnancies may be related to maternal factors associated with infertility rather than the type of assisted reproductive technology procedure used. *Fertil Steril.* 2012 Oct;98(4):922–928. PubMed PMID: 22763098.

55. Ishihara O, Araki R, Kuwahara A, Itakura A, Saito H, Adamson GD. Impact of frozen-thawed single-blastocyst transfer on maternal and neonatal outcome: An analysis of 277,042 single-embryo transfer cycles from 2008 to 2010 in Japan. *Fertil Steril.* 2014 Jan;101(1):128–133. PubMed PMID: 24268706.

56. Wikland M, Hardarson T, Hillensjo T et al. Obstetric outcomes after transfer of vitrified blastocysts. *Hum Reprod.* 2010 Jul;25(7):1699–1707. PubMed PMID: 20472913.

2

Pathophysiology of Accreta

Eric Jauniaux, Amar Bhide, and Graham J. Burton

CONTENTS

Introduction

Placenta accreta (PA) is a relatively new disorder of human placentation. In 1937, Irving and Hertig published what was to become the classical study of PA.[1] They defined PA as the abnormal adherence either in whole or in part of "the afterbirth" to the underlying uterine wall and suggested that the pathological basis of PA is the complete or partial absence of the decidua basalis. Although their series of 20 cases included only superficial PA, also called PA vera, they describe placenta increta as instances where the chorionic villi penetrate deeply into the uterine wall and placenta percreta where the villi perforates the entire uterus. Interestingly, only one case in their series had a previous history of caesarean delivery (CD). Similarly, in their literature review up to 1935, only one out of 106 cases had a previous CD and a previous manual removal of the placenta or uterine curettage amounted to more 95% of the possible etiologies of PA in subsequent pregnancies. By contrast, in 1966 when Luke et al. published their series of PA, 9 of their 21 cases had a previous history of CD.[2]

Until the 19th century, the caesarean section (CS) was a surgical procedure of last resort performed almost exclusively to save the baby's life.[3] It is only when surgeons started to suture the uterus after delivery that the maternal death rate started to improve. Further major technical advances in the surgical technique in the 20th century substantially reduced the complication rates of CD. As a consequence, mothers not only increasingly survived the surgical procedure but were also able to have one or more subsequent pregnancies. Changes in PA incidence secondary to changes in CD rates are often delayed by one or two decades, depending on the interval between pregnancies and birth rates, which may vary in different part of world. Over the last 40 years, there has been an exponential increase in the rates of CD from less than 10% to over 30% and a 10-fold rise in the incidence of PA in most high income countries. In the last decade, the rates of CD have also increased exponentially in middle and low-income countries with countries like Egypt and Turkey reaching rates of 50%. All recent epidemiologic studies have shown a clear association between the increase in CD rates and the incidence of PA in subsequent pregnancies. It has been recently estimated that if the CD rate continues to rise as it has in recent years in the United States, by 2020 there will be an additional 4,504 cases of PA and 130 maternal deaths due to placenta previa and PA complications annually.[4]

PA is not exclusively a consequence of CD, curettage, or manual removal of the placenta. Any form of damage, even small, to the integrity of the uterine lining has been associated with PA in subsequent pregnancies. Causes include surgical abortions, insertion of an intrauterine device, myomectomy, chemotherapy, and radiation.[5–7] More recently hysteroscopic surgery, endometrial resection, and uterine artery embolization have been found to be associated with subsequent PA.[8] Interestingly, IVF procedures,[9–12] which may be linked to a small trauma to the endometrium, and uterine pathology, such as bicornuate uterus, adenomyosis, submucous fibroids,[5–7,13] or myotonic dystrophy,[14] which indirectly affect the structure of the uterus, have also been associated with subsequent PA. Endometritis can lead to endometrial fibrosis and poor decidualization and was found as a possible cause of abnormally adherent placenta;[1] it has become an uncommon cause of PA with the use of antibiotics.

Histopathologically, PA is now universally defined by a partial or complete absence of decidua basalis resulting in placental villi being attached to or invading the scarred myometrium underneath.[1,2,5–7] PA has also been subdivided into total, partial, or focal, depending on the amount of placental tissue involved.[1] Luke et al.[2] criticized this classification on the basis that the degree of penetration of the uterine wall is not uniform and that histological examination of the placenta is rarely complete and often distorted by attempts at manual removal. In the last decade, PA has been increasingly being referred to as "morbidly adherent" placenta (MAP), by obstetricians and ultrasonographers. This terminology which was only used by nineteenth-century physicians to describe a retained placenta is confusing as it refers to a placenta that is superficially adherent to the uterine wall without invasion of the myometrium by chorionic villi. Difficulty in manually removing the placenta after a birth with excessive bleeding is often perceived by clinicians as being due to abnormal placental adherence and thus classified as accreta. Thus epidemiological data and prenatal imaging studies based on clinical diagnosis without histopathological confirmation of PA can only overestimate the true prevalence of PA. The subdivision of PA into abnormally adherent (accreta vera) and abnormally invasive (increta or percreta) is essential for the diagnosis and management of PA, and many series have included a mixed bag of cases with various degrees of chorionic villi invasion of the myometrium. Further studies should clearly separate the two conditions and include a detailed pathological examination correlated with prenatal imaging features in each case.

Although the risk factors for PA are well known, the underlying mechanisms leading to abnormal adherence or invasive placentation are less well understood. Both the decidua and the myometrium play a role in the development of PA. This chapter reviews the pathophysiology of PA and evaluates the possible mechanisms leading to an abnormally invasion of the uterine wall by placental tissue.

The Uterine Scar Effect

On the anterior uterine wall of the uterine corpus, the muscle fibers from each side crisscross diagonally with those of the opposite side but run in a predominantly transverse direction.[15,16] Laterally, the fibers are not completely parallel and they overlap, whereas muscle fibers run in an anterior and posterior direction over the fundus of the uterus. The cervical wall is made up of dense connective tissue with only around 10% of smooth muscle fibers (Figure 2.1).

The main anatomical impact of a uterine surgical procedure such as a CS or a myomectomy will be at the level of smooth muscular layers of the myometrium. The first "modern" CS deliveries were performed using a vertical incision for both the abdomen and uterine entry.[3] The "lower segment" transverse CS is now the most commonly performed procedure for CS deliveries around the world. The so-called "classical" vertical uterine incision does much more damage to the myometrium and is at higher risk of spontaneous uterine rupture in subsequent pregnancies than the transverse lower segment incision. It is therefore only used in rare cases of very early preterm birth (23–25 weeks), the delivery of the fetus in cases of placenta previa accreta, and for the delivery of conjoined twins.[17]

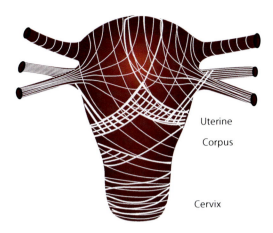

Uterine

Corpus

Cervix

FIGURE 2.1   Diagram of the uterine corpus showing the muscle fibers from each side crisscross diagonally with those of the opposite side.

Postsurgical Uterine Healing

Ferdinand Kehrer (1837–1914) and Max Sänger (1853–1903) each independently developed uterine closure methods using sutures made of silver wire, as utilized successfully by the American gynecologist James Marion Sims (1813–1883) to repair vesico-vaginal fistulae.[3] Most surgeons now use synthetic absorbable braided sutures with polyglycolic acid, polycaprolactone, and calcium stearate coating or polyglycolic sutures, while chromic catgut is avoided. All have different properties, which can potentially have an impact on the healing process.

Many surgeons of the first half of the 20th century have speculated that "correct" approximation of the cut margins, that is, decidua-to-decidua, myometrium to myometrium, serosa to serosa, would not result in any thinning of lower segment after CD, and thus the uterus would be able to withstand the stress of labor in future. Schwarz, for example, concluded that if the cut surfaces are closely apposed, the proliferation of the connective tissue is minimal, and the normal relation of the smooth muscle to connective tissue in gradually reestablished.[18] Williams found that at the time of repeat CD the exterior of the uterus revealed no trace of a previous incision and believed that the uterus heals by regeneration of the muscular fibers and not by scar tissue.[19]

Muscles in general, and the myometrium in particular, do not actually heal by regenerating muscle fibers, but by forming "foreign" substances including collagen. The resulting scar tissue is weaker, less elastic, and more prone to injury and dehiscence (separation) than the intact muscle. Myofiber disarray, tissue edema, inflammation, and elastosis have all been observed in uterine wound healing after surgery.[20] Experiments in mice have also indicated that differences in regenerative ability translate into histological, proliferative, and functional differences in biomechanical properties of the scarred myometrium after CD.[21] These results could explain the wide individual variations observed in uterine healing after CD.

Uterine Scar and Defects

When suturing the uterus during the closing phase of a CD, the primary aim of the surgeon is to stop the bleeding from the edges of the uterine incision. This can often be achieved with one layer of suture.[17] Max Sänger was the first to advocate in 1882 a two-layer uterine closure for CD surgical procedures.[3] The advantages and disadvantages of single- versus double-layer myometrium closure have remained the topic of a continuous debate ever since. Overall, single-layer closure compared with double-layer closure of the uterine incision is associated with a statistically significant reduction in mean blood loss and duration of the operative procedure.[17] A large multicenter, case-control study has shown that a prior single-layer closure carries more than twice the risk of uterine rupture compared with double-layer closure.[22] A systematic review of the best available evidence regarding the association between single-layer closure and uterine rupture in women attempting a vaginal birth after a previous CD found that locked, but not unlocked, single-layer closures are associated with a higher uterine rupture risk than double-layer closure.[23] A small retrospective study also found that the use of monofilament suture for hysterotomy closure in prior CS significantly reduces the chance of having placenta previa and thus PA in the index pregnancy.[24]

Single-layer closure and locked first layer are possibly coupled with thinner residual myometrium thickness.[25] A small randomized clinical trial (RCT) of single versus double layer on uterine healing, evaluated by assessed by hydrosonography 6 months after cesarean delivery, has indicated that a double-layer locked/unlocked closure of the uterine incision decreases the risk of poor uterine scar healing.[26] A recent retrospective cohort study using transvaginal ultrasound found that residual myometrial thickness is greater and scar defect length, but not depth and width, is smaller following double-layer compared with single-layer closure.[27] A recent case-control study has found that continuous sutures on the inner side of the uterine wall increases the risks of development of PA in subsequent pregnancies presenting with placenta previa.[28]

Simple and multiple CD scars can be accurately identified with transvaginal sonography (TVS), many years after the last surgical procedure (Figure 2.2). A uterine caesarean delivery defect (CDD) or "niche" is a larger and deeper defect of the myometrium. A CDD may range from a small defect of the superficial myometrium (Figure 2.3) to a wide and deep defect with clear loss of substance from the endometrial cavity down to the uterine serosa (Figure 2.4). In women with a history of previous CD, CD scar defects have been found to range between 20% and 65% of the wall thickness on transvaginal ultrasound.[29-33] The risk of scar deficiency/separation, where the defect involves the deep myometrial layers, is increased in women with a retroflexed uterus, in those who have undergone multiple CDs, and after CD in advanced labour.[29] Large CDD could explain rare reports of placenta percreta leading to uterine rupture in the first half of pregnancy.[34-38] Although this is an extremely rare complication of placentation, the mechanism of uterine rupture due to a placenta percreta is likely to be similar to that of a tubal rupture in an ectopic placentation. There is potential for the formation of abnormal vascular communications between artery and vein during the healing process of a uterine scar,[39] and this has recently been associated with the development of PA.[40] These findings emphasize the pivotal role of the superficial myometrium in modulating normal placentation. Placental tissue implanting into a CDD can probably lead more often to placenta percreta and uterine rupture. However, this will remain a hypothesis until we obtain data from prospective studies on the size of a CDD and the risk of PA in subsequent pregnancies.

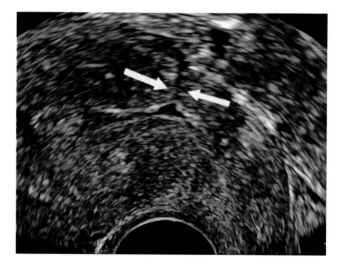

FIGURE 2.2 Transvaginal ultrasound view of the uterus in a nonpregnant woman with a history of two previous caesarean deliveries (CDs), 7 and 9 years before the examination. Note the small defect through the uterine wall at the junction between the lower and upper uterine segment (arrows) corresponding to the scar of the CD incision.

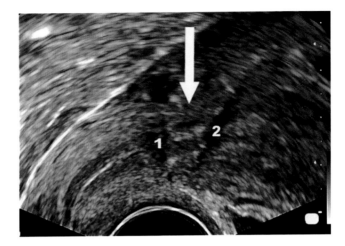

FIGURE 2.3 Transvaginal ultrasound view of the uterus in a nonpregnant woman with a history of two previous CDs (1st emergent and 2nd elective). Note the two small defects (1 and 2) through the uterine wall at the junction between the lower and upper uterine segment (arrow) corresponding to the scar of the caesarean section (CS) incisions.

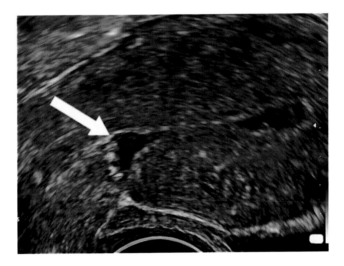

FIGURE 2.4 Transvaginal ultrasound 3D view of the uterus in a nonpregnant woman with a history of a previous emergency CD showing a large defect at the junction between lower and upper uterine segment (arrow) connecting the endometrial cavity with the visceral serosa.

Scar Pregnancies

A caesarean scar pregnancy is the implantation of clinically detectable pregnancy into a scar. It can be recurrent and is associated with severe maternal morbidity and significant mortality from very early in pregnancy.[41] It has been suggested that a caesarean pregnancy is not a separate entity from PA but rather a continuum of the same condition.[42,43] However, not all scar pregnancies require major surgery or lifesaving hysterectomy at the time of delivery,[44] suggesting that in some cases the scar defect can be large enough to host an entire gestational sac without the villi of the definitive placenta implanting deep into the myometrium. A small recent prospective study of transvaginal ultrasound of CD scar 14–16 weeks after delivery has indicated that both elective and emergent low segment incision are associated with scars involving the cervix.[45] The cervical wall is essentially made up of connective tissue with only 10% of smooth muscle fibers. This can probably explain why cervical scar pregnancies are more symptomatic and almost always lead to major bleeding early in pregnancy. These data suggest that a scar pregnancy does not systematically lead to villous tissue entering the myometrium, but depending on the size and location of the scar defect, the symptoms of an accreta and a non-accreta scar pregnancy can be very similar. The diagnosis of PA can only be confirmed by the histological examination of a total hysterectomy or partial resection specimen, and thus in cases of successful conservative management it is difficult to be certain that scar pregnancy was truly accreta.

The scars of surgical abortions, insertion of an intrauterine device, and uterine curettages should not be associated with major secondary damage to the myometrium, but they have all been associated with PA.[5–7] Fragments of myometrium are found in the products of conception in around a third of surgical terminations and uterine curettage for miscarriage.[46] Myometrial fibers have also been found in the basal plate in a placenta from a previous delivery in women presenting with PA, and greater quantities of myometrial fibers in a delivered placenta are significantly associated with the subsequent development of accreta.[47] The fact that there is no clear correlation between superficial myometrial damage and PA in a subsequent pregnancy suggests that the trauma to the myometrium and the surface of the endometrial damage is often limited in a curettage procedure compared to that of a CS. If the myometrium scar is small, the placenta will simply grow over it, which can explain why the majority of placenta previa in cases of a previous CD are not accreta. Only large prospective cohort multicentric studies will be able to provide the answer to the relationship between the location and extent of myometrium damage after uterine surgery and the risk of PA in subsequent pregnancies.

The Accreta Placenta

Several concepts have been proposed to explain why and how PA occurs. The oldest concept is based on a theoretical primary defect of trophoblast biology leading to excessive invasion of the myometrium. The other prevailing hypothesis is that of a secondary defect of the endometrial–myometrial interface leading to a failure of normal decidualization in the area of the uterine scar allowing an abnormally deep PV anchoring and trophoblast infiltration (Figure 2.5).

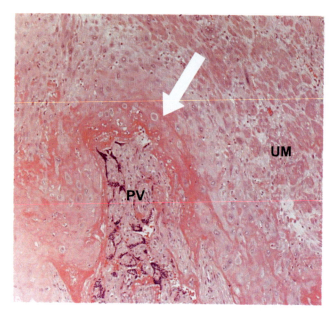

FIGURE 2.5   Microscopic view of accreta (arrow) placental villi (PV) within the uterine myometrium (UM). H&E × 10. (Courtesy of Dr. Lona Jeffrey.)

Normal Implantation and Placentation

During the secretory phase of the menstrual cycle, the endometrium transforms into well-vascularized receptive tissue, which is characterized by the proliferation and differentiation of the stromal cells into decidual cells, the infiltration of maternal immune cells, and vascular remodeling of the endometrial vessels.[48,49] In the first trimester, migratory leucocytes account for 30% of the endometrial cells, and of those 75% are uterine natural killer (uNK) cells of the maternal innate immune system.[50] Vascular changes of the deciduas include induction of angiogenesis, vascular permeability, and arterial remodeling.[49] Decidualization of the endometrium is essential for implantation and normal placental development. The process is complex and involves many local uterine components and external maternal cells and hormones. Decidualized stromal cells are derived from the fibroblast-like cells within the endometrium, which maintain their progesterone receptors in the presence of progesterone. Progesterone also initiates the proliferation on endometrial glands from before the blastocyst implants.[51] Secretions from the uterine glands appear critical for uterine receptivity and blastocyst implantation. The secretions also represent an important source of nutrients, histotroph, for the conceptus during the first trimester.[52,53]

The formative stages of human placental development are largely unknown because of their existence in a "black box" where access to samples is extremely limited for ethical reasons.[54] Implantation relies on the interaction of the trophectoderm cells forming the wall of the blastocyst with the cells uterine epithelium. On establishing contact, some of the trophectoderm cells undergo proliferation and fusion to from the multinucleated syncytiotrophoblast, whereas others remain as a deeper, progenitor population, the cytotrophoblast cells. Tongues of syncytiotrophoblast penetrate between the epithelial cells, while at the same time the endometrial stromal cells grow over and encapsulate the conceptus. The combination of these actions leads to the conceptus soon becoming completely embedded within the stratum compactum of the endometrium. Soon after, strands of mononuclear cytotrophoblast start to proliferate at the fetal side of the implanted blastocyst wall.[54–56] The resulting cytotrophoblastic columns push themselves into the primitive syncytiotrophoblastic mass to form early villi. The most distal cytotrophoblast cells break through the syncytium and spread laterally to form the cytotrophoblastic shell separating the placenta from the decidua. Cells on the outer surface of the shell differentiate into nonproliferative, cytotrophoblast cells that invade the decidual stroma, collectively called extravillous trophoblast (EVT). They differentiate primarily into interstitial and endovascular subpopulations that migrate through the decidual stroma and down the lumens of the spiral arteries, respectively. The interstitial EVTs invade the uterine wall as far as the inner third of the uterine myometrium (UM),[55,56] where they fuse to form multinucleated trophoblast giant cells.[57] EVT cells can first be found both within and around the spiral arteries in the central area of the placenta. They gradually extend laterally, reaching the periphery of the placenta around midgestation. Depthwise, the changes are maximal within the central region of the placental bed, and the extent of invasion is progressively shallower toward the periphery. The EVTs physically anchor the primitive placenta to the decidua. The endovascular cells also act as plugs blocking the spiral arteries and preventing maternal blood flow from entering the intervillous space during the first 10–12 weeks of gestation.[58] This phenomenon creates an environment of physiological hypoxia inside the gestational sac, which is essential for normal placenta and fetal development to occur.[59,60]

Both endovascular and interstitial EVT invasion are associated with the physiological conversion of the terminal part of the uterine circulation down to the basal part of the spiral arteries at level of the junctional zone (JZ) of the inner third of the myometrium.[56,61] The EVT cells penetrate the JZ via the action of their proteases on the intercellular ground substance, affecting its mechanical and electrophysiological properties and those of spiral arteries changing the structure of their wall. In addition, activation of the uNK cells through immune interactions with the EVT is thought to release further proteases and cytokines in the immediate vicinity of the spiral arteries that contribute to the remodeling. Insufficient activation of the maternal immune cells is associated with complications of pregnancy, including miscarriage, preeclampsia, and growth restriction.[62] The remodeling of the spiral arteries is characterized by the progressive loss of myocytes from their media and their internal elastic lamina, which are replaced by fibrinoid material.[56] Consequently, these vessels lose their responsiveness to circulating vasoactive compounds and become a low-resistance vascular network by dilatation.[58] This transformation, termed "physiological changes," results in the metamorphosis of small caliber spiral vessels into flaccid distended arteries with a 5- to 10-fold dilation at the vessel mouth. The uNK cells and macrophages seem to prime vessels for EVT invasion and play a role in recruiting EVT cells to temporarily reline vessels wall before the maternal endothelium regrows.[49] Around 30–50 spiral arteries are transformed during the first trimester. In normal pregnancies, the transformation of spiral arteries into utero-placental arteries is described as completed around midgestation.[58] However, there is a gradient in the infiltration of the EVTs along the spiral artery, and even in normal pregnancy not all spiral arteries are completely transformed.[56,63]

In humans, it is obvious that the decidua does not act as barrier but rather as a passageway for EVT cells to colonize the JZ in a regulated manner. Trophoblast invasion is notably more aggressive and more penetrative at sites of ectopic implantation, for example, in the Fallopian tube, in the absence of decidua. As the EVT differentiate they progressively display a more migratory phenotype, changing their integrin repertoire from predominantly collagen IV receptors to fibronectin and then laminin receptors.[64] At the same time, they increase their expression of members of the matrix metalloproteinases (MMPs) family. Of these, most attention has been paid to the gelatinases, MMP-2 and MMP-9, that break down native collagen IV and denatured collagens. Both are secreted by the EVT but require cleavage by membrane-bound MMPs, such as MMP-14 and -15 for activation, adding complexity to the situation. Evidence suggests that MMP-2 is most significant early in pregnancy, but that MMP-9 becomes more important toward the end of the first trimester.[65] Other pathways potentially underpinning trophoblast invasion include the plasminogen activator system. The urokinase-type plasminogen activator receptor (uPAR) has been immunolocalized to EVT[66] and on activation cleaves plasminogen to plasmin. Plasmin could assist in either breakdown of the extracellular matrix or cleavage of pro-MMPs. In addition, EVTs express high levels of the cysteine cathepsin protease, cathepsin L,[67] and the ADAM family of peptidases has also recently been implicated.[68] An array of factors operate upstream of these pathways to stimulate trophoblast invasion.[6,48,49] Identification of these has largely been based on in vitro assays of invasion into artificial matrices by trophoblast-like cell lines or explant cultures of early PV, and caution should be exercised when extrapolating the data to the in vivo state. Nonetheless, they include cytokines and growth factors, such as epidermal growth factor, vascular endothelial growth factor (VEGF), interleukin-1β, tumor necrosis factor-α, and the hyperglycoslyated form of human chorionic gonadotropin (hCG); and hormones, such as triiodothyronine, leptin, and gonadotropin-releasing hormone-1 and low (1%) oxygen concentrations.[6]

Equally important in the regulation of placentation are the inhibitors of trophoblast invasion. Activity of the MMPs is regulated by their natural antagonists, the tissue inhibitors of metalloproteinases (TIMPs). Specificity of members of the TIMP family varies; TIMP-1 inhibits all MMPs, TIMP-2 preferentially inhibits MMP-2, and TIMP-3 antagonizes MMP-9 and MMP-14. The TIMPs immunolocalize to the EVT[69] and are capable of inhibiting invasion in vitro.[70] Similarly, the urokinase plasminogen activator (uPA) system may be modulated by plasminogen activator inhibitor PAI-1.[71] Factors favoring inhibition of invasion in vitro include transforming growth factor-β, interleukin-10, leukemia inhibitory factor, progesterone, kisspeptin-10, and 3% oxygen compared to 20%.[72–74] Low oxygen concentrations tend to stimulate EVT proliferation and VEGF messenger RNA expression, while ambient levels have an inhibitory effect.

The precise regulation of trophoblast invasion will therefore depend on the balance of local concentrations of many factors and also the composition of the extracellular matrix. For example, collagen type IV (col-IV), which is a structural protein providing tissue integrity, has recently been shown to influence the invasive behavior of EVT cells at the implantation site.[75] However, it is clear that the repertoire of proteinases expressed by the EVT provides them with the necessary molecular machinery to break down scar tissue present in the uterus.

Although much has been learned about the how invasion may be modulated at the molecular level, one of the big unanswered questions at present is what stops the EVT from penetrating further than the inner third of the myometrium in normal pregnancies. Having passed through the decidua the cells are now largely beyond the reach of the maternal immune cells. Is it lack of stimulation that brings them to a halt, or is there a strong local inhibitory signal? Equally, is fusion associated with loss of invasiveness, and if so, it is cause or consequence? Answers to these and other related questions are just as important in the context of PA as knowing what stimulates EVT invasion in the first place, and yet they have not received the equivalent research attention.

The Scarred Decidua

Total or partial absence of decidua with villous tissue below the JZ is the pathognomonic histological feature of PA at delivery.[7] The increased incidence of placenta previa after a previous CS[4,13,23] supports the concept of a biologically defective decidua rather than a primarily abnormally invasive trophoblast.[7] However, a recent meta-analysis of five cohort and 11 case-control studies published between 1990 and 2011 has indicated that after a CD, the calculated summary odds ratios (OR) are 1.47 for placenta previa and 1.96 for PA.[76] Large cohort studies in the United States have indicated an overall incidence of PA of one in 533 deliveries.[4] A case-controlled study has suggested that women with a primary elective CS without labor are more likely to develop PA in a subsequent pregnancy with placenta previa, compared with those undergoing primary emergent CS with labor.[77] Thus, PA remains a relatively uncommon obstetric pathology, suggesting that a uterine scar does not systemically lead to placenta previa, which does not automatically lead to PA.

A recent study of the uterine circulation in women with a previous CS has shown that the uterine artery resistance is increased and the volume of uterine blood flow is decreased as a fraction of maternal cardiac output compared to women with a previous vaginal birth.[78] The finding of leukocyte recruitment to the endometrium during the secretory phase following a CS[79] supports the hypothesis of abnormal decidualization in PA. Overall, these data suggest a possible relationship between a poorly vascularized uterine scar area and an increase in the resistance to blood flow in the uterine circulation with a secondary impact on reepithelialization of the scar area and defective subsequent decidualization. Individual wound healing characteristics may predispose to deep invasion of the placental bed by the EVT in PA.

The Accreta Trophoblast

The trophoblast at the maternal–placental interface in PA has been reported to be different at delivery (Table 2.1) from the more usual placental bed multinucleated giant cells (MNGCs) found in normal placentation.[80–84] Histopathological studies have found that in PA many EVTs are hypertrophic and that their numbers are increased.[82,84] The EVTs appear as a thickened band at the implantation site, and confluence is also more frequent in PA. By contrast, the number of MNGCs is reduced in the basal decidua of women with PA. It is not clear from these observations whether the EVTs are genuinely hyperplastic since cell densities rather than total numbers are reported. The proliferative index and apoptotic rate are similar to normally implanted placentas,[82,84] and so it may be that the normal number of EVT is packed into a smaller volume of decidua.

TABLE 2.1

Histopathological and Immunostaining Changes Observed in PA

- Increase in the size, numbers, and depth of myometrial invasion of EVT cells
- Reduced numbers of placental bed MNGCs
- Chorionic villi invasion of myometrial vascular spaces
- Increased labeling for EGFR in syncytiotrophoblastic cells
- Lower immunostaining for EGF c-(erbB-2), VEGFR-2 and endothelial cell tyrosine kinase receptor Tie-2 in syncytiotrophoblastic cells
- Increased VEGF and phosphotyrosine immunostaining in EVT cells
- Lower immunostaining sFLT-1 in EVT cells

Abbreviations: EGFR, epidermal growth factor receptor; EVT, extravillous trophoblast; MNGC, multinucleated giant cell; sFLT-1, soluble fms-like tyrosine kinase 1; VEGF, vascular endothelial growth factor; VEGFR-2, vascular endothelial growth factor receptor 2.

Stronger labeling for epidermal growth factor receptor (EGFR) and lower staining for EGF c-(erbB-2), VEGFR-2, and endothelial cell tyrosine kinase receptor Tie-2 in the villous syncytiotrophoblast have also been reported in PA.[85–88] Increased syncytiotrophoblast EGFR in PA suggest that abnormal villous adherence develops as a result of abnormal expression of growth-, angiogenesis-, and invasion-related factors in trophoblast populations (Table 2.1). Difference in cellular receptor expression between the villous syncytiotrophoblast, which has no invasive capacity, and the invasive EVT in PA is difficult to interpret. Similarly, lower maternal serum (MS) levels of free-beta human chorionic gonadotrophin (fβhCG) and higher levels of pregnancy-associated plasma protein A (PAPP-A) in PA compared to both normal controls and cases of placenta previa[89] are difficult to explain. Both hormones are essentially produced by the syncytiotrophoblast and reflect its expansion, but no difference in either placental or fetal growth pattern has been reported in abnormally adherent placentas.

Ki-67, a nuclear protein that is associated with, and may be necessary for, cellular proliferation is rarely observed in EVT, except in the trophoblast columns of first-trimester PA cases.[90] Increased VEGF and phosphotyrosine immunostaining has been observed in EVT cells from PA.[91] These cells also co-expressed vimentin and cytokeratin-7, an epithelial-to-mesenchymal transition feature and tumor-like cell phenotype (Table 2.1). Lower MS levels of free VEGF and a switch of the interstitial EVT to a metastable cell phenotype have been reported in placenta previa with excessive myometrial invasion.[91] One of the proposed mechanisms through which the EVTs lose their invasive phenotype is through syncytial-type fusion into MNGCs.[90] The secretion of VEGF by MNGCs is likely to be one of the signals initiating and coordinating vascularization in the decidua and placenta during implantation.[92] More recently, soluble fms-like tyrosine kinase (sFLT-1), which is a potent antiangiogenic growth factor that has been found to be markedly elevated in preeclampsia, has been found in lower concentration in the MS and in lower immunostaining in the EVTs cells of women presenting with PA.[93] These findings suggest that VEGF and sFLT-1 play a pivotal role in the process of pathological programming of EVTs toward increased motility and invasiveness in PA.

Absent JZ Myometrium and Deep Uterine Vasculature Remodeling

EVTs invade the uterine wall to a significantly greater depth in PA.[90] Placenta increta and percreta are not due to a further invasion of EVT in the uterine wall. They are likely to arise secondary to dehiscence of a scar, leading to the presence of chorionic villi deep within the uterine wall, and thus give EVTs greater access to the deep myometrium. Deeper trophoblast myometrial invasion and chorionic villi infiltration into myometrial vascular spaces has been recently documented in placenta increta and percreta.[94] This leads to absence of the normal plane of cleavage above the decidua basalis, thus preventing placental separation after delivery in cases of PA (Figure 2.6), and can explain the higher level of cell-free placental mRNA in these cases.[95,96]

Numbers of interstitial EVTs are increased in PA[94] but spiral artery remodeling is reduced, more so in PA cases without local decidua,[80,83] and is sometimes completely absent in the accreta area.[80] This is in contrast with the reduction in trophoblast invasion and failure of conversion of the spiral arteries, which accompanies common complications of pregnancy, such as preeclampsia and fetal growth restriction and suggests a different pathophysiologic mechanism. It may be that in the absence of a decidua, the normal release of proteases and cytokines from activated maternal immune cells is missing, impairing arterial remodeling. Invasion of larger vessels in the outer myometrium and near the serosa in PA is probably determined by access rather than a preexisting defect in trophoblastic growth that would produce uncontrolled invasion of EVT through the entire depth of the myometrium,[90] transforming the arterial vasculature beyond the level of the JZ.[7] Excessive dilatation of the arcuate arteries is the most prominent feature of PA prenatally on ultrasound and macroscopically on the uterine surface at delivery (Figure 2.7). The sonographic finding of intraplacental blood "lacunae" in placenta increta and percreta appears to be due to supply from larger, deeper vessels than seen in normal implantation, transformed by endovascular EVT.[97]

The comparison of ultrasound features of uterine caesarean scar with histological findings has shown that large and deep myometrial defects are often associated with absence of reepithelialization

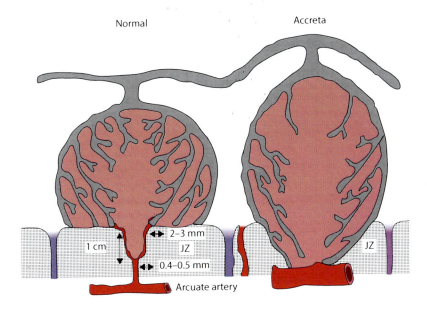

FIGURE 2.6 Diagram showing a normal and an accreta placental cotyledon. Note the accreta villi reaching the arcuate artery through the junctional zone (JZ) of the inner third of the myometrium, the dilatation of the arcuate circulation, and the absence of a cleavage zone.

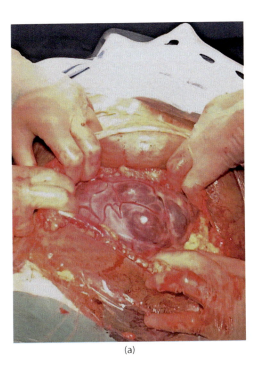

(a)

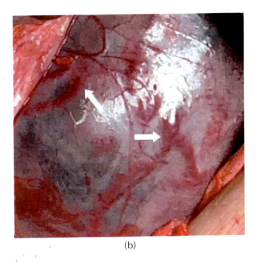

(b)

FIGURE 2.7 (a) Macroscopic view of the uterus at the level of the placentation site in a case of placenta accreta (PA). (b) The uterine wall is almost transparent and area of the abnormally implanted villous tissue is very thin and friable and surrounded by dilated vascular channels (arrows). (Courtesy of Dr. Edwin Chandraharan.)

of the scar area.[79] These findings emphasize the role of the subdecidual myometrium in modulating placentation and its replacement by scar tissue in secondary dysfunctional decidualization and trophoblastic over-invasiveness. The absence of decidua in first-trimester cases of PA negates previous suggestions that decidua is normal at the beginning of gestation and atrophies as pregnancy proceeds.[90]

Clinical–Pathological Correlations

Ultrasound imaging and magnetic resonance imaging (MRI) are now commonly used for the prenatal diagnosis of PA. Many imaging studies do not include a pathological confirmation of accreta or when they do it is limited to a brief description of number of cases that were examined without a precise description of extent of the placental attachment, degree of invasion, or spatial relationship of the accreta tissue with the previous CD scar, cervix, and so on. A recent systematic review has found that the wide heterogeneity in terminology used to describe the grades of accreta placentation and differences in study design limits the evaluation of the accuracy of ultrasound imaging in the screening and diagnosis of PA.[98] Dannheim et al.[99] have recently proposed methods of gross dissection, microscopic examination, and reporting of hysterectomy specimens containing PA. Their protocol facilitates retrospective correlation with surgical and imaging findings as well as standardized tissue sampling for potential research. Similarly, the international Abnormally Invasive Placenta (AIP) Expert Group has proposed a classification of the sonographic features of PA on both grayscale and color Doppler ultrasound imaging.[100] Distinguishing abnormally adherent from invasive placenta and percreta from increta may be difficult due to intraoperative disruption or not be possible in cases of conservative management. Correlation of pathological findings with the clinical notes and imaging is essential. It is therefore necessary that these protocols are standardized and used by both clinicians and pathologists to improve the diagnostic accuracy of radiologic imaging and the perinatal management of PA.

Conclusions

The strongest risk factor for placenta previa and PA is a prior CD indicating that a failure of decidualization in the area of a previous uterine scar can have an impact on both implantation and placentation. These findings suggest that the decidual defect following the artificial creation of a scar in the UM has an adverse effect on early implantation by creating conditions for preferential attachment of the blastocyst to scar tissue and facilitating abnormally deep invasion of the EVT.

What happens during the initial phase of placentation in PA remains a mystery. We can only witness the consequences of an abnormally deep trophoblast migration and villous attachment below the JZ at delivery. Histopathologic data support the concept that the morphological changes observed in the EVT in PA are environmental, and thus the consequence of an unusual and prolonged interaction of the EVT with the highly vascularized deep myometrium which these cells would normally not reach in normal uterine placentation.

Overall, these findings support the concept of a primary deciduo-myometrium defect in PA, exposing the myometrium and the uterine vasculature below the JZ to the migrating trophoblast. The loss of this normal plane of cleavage and the excessive vascular remodeling of the radial and arcuate arteries can explain the prenatal ultrasound findings and the clinical consequence of PA.

Macroscopic and microscopic examinations of hysterectomy specimens or myometrial samples from an abnormal placentation site remain the gold standard of reference to confirm the diagnosis of PA. Correlation of the ultrasound imaging from early in pregnancy with histopathological examination is pivotal to better understand the natural evolution of this disorder and further collaborative research is essential to improve the diagnosis and management of this increasingly common major obstetric complication.

REFERENCES

1. Irving C, Hertig AT. A study of placenta accreta. Surgery. *Gynecol Obstet.* 1937;64:178–200.
2. Luke RK, Sharpe JW, Greene RR. Placenta accreta: The adherent or invasive placena. *Am J Obstet Gynecol.* 1966;95:660–668.
3. West MJ, Irvine LM, Jauniaux E. Caesarean section: From antiquity to the 21st century. In: Jauniaux E, Grobman W, eds. *A Textbook of Caesarean Section.* Oxford: Oxford University Press; 2016:9–24.
4. Solheim KN, Esakoff TF, Little SE, Cheng YW, Sparks TN, Caughey AB. The effect of cesarean delivery rates on the future incidence of placenta previa, placenta accreta, and maternal mortality. *J Matern Fetal Neonatal Med.* 2011;24:1341–1346.
5. Fox H. Abnormalities of placentation. In: *Pathology of the Placenta,* 2nd Ed. London: Saunders; 1997:54–76.
6. Benirschke K, Burton GJ, Baergen RN. Nonvillous parts and trophoblast invasion. In: Benirschke K, Burton GJ, Baergen RN, eds. *Pathology of the Human Placenta,* 6th Ed. New York: Springer; 2012:157–240.
7. Jauniaux E, Jurkovic D. Placenta accreta: Pathogenesis of a 20th century iatrogenic uterine disease. *Placenta.* 2012;33:244–251.
8. Kanter G, Packard L, Sit AS. Placenta accreta in a patient with a history of uterine artery embolization for postpartum hemorrhage. *J Perinatol.* 2013;33:482–483.
9. Esh-Broder E, Ariel I, Abas-Bashir N et al. Placenta accreta is associated with IVF pregnancies: A retrospective chart review. *BJOG.* 20 11;118:1084–1089.
10. Hayashi M, Nakai A, Satoh S, Matsuda Y. Adverse obstetric and perinatal outcomes of singleton pregnancies may be related to maternal factors associated with infertility rather than the type of assisted reproductive technology procedure used. *Fertil Steril.* 2012;98:922–928.
11. Ishihara O, Araki R, Kuwahara A et al. Impact of frozen-thawed single-blastocyst transfer on maternal and neonatal outcome: An analysis of 277,042 single-embryo transfer cycles from 2008 to 2010 in Japan. *Fertil Steril.* 2014;101:128–133
12. Kaser DJ, Melamed A, Bormann CL et al. Cryopreserved embryo transfer is an independent risk factor for placenta accreta. *Fertil Steril.* 2015;103: 1176–1184.
13. Wu S, Kocherginsky M, Hibbard JU. Abnormal placentation: Twenty-year analysis. *Am J Obstet Gynecol.* 2005;192:1458–1461.
14. Freeman RM. Placenta accreta and myotonic dystrophy: Two cases. *BJOG.* 1991;98:594–595.
15. Schwalm H, Dubrauszky V. The structure of the musculature of the human uterus—Muscles and connective tissue. *Am J Obstet Gynecol.* 1966;94:391–404.
16. Hughesdon PE. The fibromuscular structure of the cervix and its changes during pregnancy and labour. *J Obstet Gynaecol Br Commonw.* 1952;59:763–776.
17. Jauniaux E, Berghella V. The modern caesarean section. In: Jauniaux E, Grobman W, eds. *A Textbook of Caesarean Section.* Oxford: Oxford University Press; 2016:49–68.
18. Schwarz O, Paddock R, Bortnic AR. The cesarean scar: An experimental study. *Am J Obstet Gynecol.* 1938;36:962.
19. Williams JW. A critical analysis of 21 years experience with cesarean section. *Bull Johns Hopkins Hosp.* 1921;32:173.
20. Roeder HA, Cramer SF, Leppert PC. A look at uterine wound healing through a histopathological study of uterine scars. *Reprod Sci.* 2012;19:463–473.
21. Buhimschi CS, Zhao G, Sora N et al. Myometrial wound healing post-Cesarean delivery in the MRL/MpJ mouse model of uterine scarring. *Am J Pathol.* 2010;177:197–207.
22. Roberge S, Chaillet N, Boutin A et al. Single-versus double-layer closure of the hysterotomy incision during cesarean delivery and risk of uterine rupture. *Int J Gynaecol Obstet.* 2011;115:5–10.
23. Chiu TL, Sadler L, Wise MR. Placenta praevia after prior caesarean section: An exploratory case-control study. *Aust N Z J Obstet Gynaecol.* 2013;53:455–458.
24. Roberge S, Demers S, Berghella V et al. Impact of single- vs double-layer closure on adverse outcomes and uterine scar defect: A systematic review and metaanalysis. *Am J Obstet Gynecol.* 2014;211:453–460.
25. Glavind J, Madsen LD, Uldbjerg N, Dueholm M. Ultrasound evaluation of Cesarean scar after single- and double-layer uterotomy closure: A cohort study. *Ultrasound Obstet Gynecol.* 2013;42:207–212.

26. Sevket O, Ates S, Molla T et al. Hydrosonographic assessment of the effects of 2 different suturing techniques on healing of the uterine scar after cesarean delivery. *Int J Gynaecol Obstet.* 2014;125: 219–222.
27. Bujold E, Goyet M, Marcoux S . The role of uterine closure in the risk of uterine rupture. *Obstet Gynecol.* 2010;116:43–50.
28. Sumigama S, Sugiyama C, Kotani T et al. Uterine sutures at prior caesarean section and placenta accreta in subsequent pregnancy: A case-control study. *BJOG.* 2014;121:866–874.
29. Ofili-Yebovi D, Ben-Nagi J, Sawyer E . Deficient lower-segment cesarean section scars: Prevalence and risk factors. *Ultrasound Obstet Gynecol.* 2008;31:72–77.
30. Wang CB, Chiu WW, Lee CY et al. Cesarean scar defect: Correlation between Cesarean section number, defect size, clinical symptoms and uterine position. *Ultrasound Obstet Gynecol.* 2009;34:85–89.
31. Chang WC, Chang DY, Huang SC et al. Use of three-dimensional ultrasonography in the evaluation of uterine perfusion and healing after laparoscopic myomectomy. *Fertil Steril.* 2009;92:1110–1115.
32. Osser OV, Jokubkiene L, Valentin L. High prevalence of defects in cesarean section scars at transvaginal ultrasound examination. *Ultrasound Obstet Gynecol.* 2009;34:90–97.
33. Jastrow N, Chaillet N, Roberge S, Morency AM, Lacasse Y, Bujold E. Sonographic lower uterine segment thickness and risk of uterine scar defect: A systematic review. *J Obstet Gynaecol Can.* 2010;32:321–327.
34. Liang HS, Jeng CJ, Sheen TC, Lee FK, Yang YC, Tzeng CR. First-trimester uterine rupture from a placenta percreta. A case report. *J Reprod Med.* 2003;489:474–478.
35. Fleisch MC, Lux J, Schoppe M et al. Placenta percreta leading to spontaneous complete uterine rupture in the second trimester. Example of a fatal complication of abnormal placentation following uterine scarring. *Gynecol Obstet Invest.* 2008;65:81–83.
36. Patsouras K, Panagopoulos P, Sioulas V et al. Uterine rupture at 17 weeks of a twin pregnancy complicated with placenta percreta. *J Obstet Gynaecol.* 2010;30:60–61.
37. Jang DG, Lee GS, Yoon JH, Lee SJ. Placenta percreta-induced uterine rupture diagnosed by laparoscopy in the first trimester. *Int J Med Sci.* 2011;8:424–427.
38. Hornemann A, Bohlmann MK, Diedrich K et al. Spontaneous uterine rupture at the 21st week of gestation caused by placenta percreta. *Arch Gynecol Obstet.* 2011;284:875–878.
39. Rygh AB, Greve OJ, Fjetland L et al. Arteriovenous malformation as a consequence of a scar pregnancy. *Acta Obstet Gynecol Scand.* 2009;88:853–855.
40. Roach MK, Thomassee MS. Acquired uterine arteriovenous malformation and retained placenta increta. *Obstet Gynecol.* 2015;126:642–644.
41. Qian ZD, Guo QY, Huang LL. Identifying risk factors for recurrent cesarean scar pregnancy: A case-control study. *Fertil Steril.* 2014;120:12 9–134.
42. Sinha P, Mishra M. Caesarean scar pregnancy: A precursor of placenta percreta/accreta. *J Obstet Gynaecol.* 2012;32:621–623.
43. Timor-Tritsch IE, Monteagudo A, Cali G et al. Cesarean scar pregnancy and early placenta accreta share common histology. *Ultrasound Obstet Gynecol.* 2014;43:383–395.
44. Jurkovic D. Caesarean scar pregnancy and placenta accreta. *Ultrasound Obstet Gynecol.* 2014;43:361–362.
45. Markovitch O, Tepper R, Hershkovitz R. Sonographic assessment of post-cesarean section uterine scar in pregnant women. *J Matern Fetal Neonatal Med.* 2013;26:173–175.
46. Beuker JM, Erwich JJ, Khong TY. Is endomyometrial injury during termination of pregnancy or curettage following miscarriage the precursor to placenta accreta? *J Clin Pathol.* 2005;58:273–275.
47. Linn RL, Miller ES, Lim G, Ernst LM. Adherent basal plate myometrial fibers in the delivered placenta as a risk factor for development of subsequent placenta accreta. *Placenta.* 2015;36:1419–1424.
48. Knöfler M. Critical growth factors and signalling pathways controlling human trophoblast invasion. *Int J Dev Biol.* 2010;54:269–280.
49. Plaisier M. Decidualisation and angiogenesis. *Best Pract Res Clin Obstet Gynaecol.* 2011;25:259–271.
50. Moffett A, Colucci F. Uterine NK cells: Active regulators at the maternal-fetal interface. *J Clin Invest.* 2014;124:1872–1879.
51. Filant J, Spencer TE. Uterine glands: Biological roles in conceptus implantation, uterine receptivity and decidualization. *Int J Dev Biol.* 2014;58:107–116.
52. Burton GJ, Jauniaux E, Charnock-Jones DS. The influence of the intrauterine environment on human placental development. *Int J Dev Biol.* 2010;54:303–312.

53. Hempstock J, Cindrova-Davies T, Jauniaux E, Burton GJ. Endometrial glands as a source of nutrients, growth factors and cytokines during the first trimester of human pregnancy: A morphological and immunohistochemical study. *Reprod Biol Endocrinol.* 2004;20:58.

54. James JL, Carter AM, Chamley LW. Human placentation from nidation to 5 weeks of gestation. Part I: What do we know about formative placental development following implantation? *Placenta.* 2012;33:327–334.

55. Pijnenborg R, Dixon G, Robertson WB, Brosens I. Trophoblastic invasion of human decidua from 8 to 18 weeks of pregnancy. *Placenta.* 1980;1:3–19.

56. Pijnenborg R, Vercruysse L, Brosens I. Deep placentation. *Best Pract Res Clin Obstet Gynaecol.* 2011;25:273–285.

57. Al-Lamki RS, Skepper JN, Burton GJ. Are human placental bed giant cells merely aggregates of small mononuclear trophoblast cells? An ultrastructural and immunocytochemical study. *Hum Reprod.* 1999;14:496–504.

58. Burton GJ, Jauniaux E, Watson AL. Maternal arterial connections to the placental intervillous space during the first trimester of human pregnancy: The Boyd collection revisited. *Am J Obstet Gynecol.* 1999;181:718–724.

59. Jauniaux E, Watson AL, Hempstock J et al. Onset of placental bloodflow and trophoblastic oxidative stress: A possible factor in human early pregnancy failure. *Am J Pathol.* 2000;157:2111–2122.

60. Jauniaux E, Poston L, Burton GJ. Placental-related diseases of pregnancy: Involvement of oxidative stress and implications in human evolution. *Hum Reprod Update.* 2006;12:747–755.

61. Burton GJ, Woods AW, Jauniaux E, Kingdom JC. Rheological and physiological consequences of conversion of the maternal spiral arteries for uteroplacental blood flow during human pregnancy. *Placenta.* 2009;30:473–482.

62. Hiby SE, Apps R, Sharkey AM et al. Maternal activating KIRs protect against human reproductive failure mediated by fetal HLA-C2. *J Clin Invest.* 2010;120:4102–4110.

63. Meekins JW, Pijnenborg R, Hanssens M et al. A study of placental bed spiral arteries and trophoblast invasion in normal and severe pre-eclamptic pregnancies. *BJOG.* 1994;101:669–674.

64. Harris LK, Jones CJ, Aplin JD. Adhesion molecules in human trophoblast—A review. II. Extravillous trophoblast. *Placenta.* 2009;30:299–304.

65. Staun-Ram E, Goldman S, Gabarin D, Shalev E. Expression and importance of matrix metalloproteinase 2 and 9 (MMP-2 and -9) in human trophoblast invasion. *Reprod Biol Endocrinol.* 2004;2:59.

66. Pierleoni C, Samuelsen GB, Graem N et al. Immunohistochemical identification of the receptor for urokinase plasminogen activator associated with fibrin deposition in normal and ectopic human placenta. *Placenta.* 1998;19:501–508.

67. Varanou A, Withington SL, Lakasing L et al. The importance of cysteine cathepsin proteases for placental development. *J Mol Med.* 2006;84:305–317.

68. Pollheimer J, Fock V, Knofler M. Review: The ADAM metalloproteinases—Novel regulators of trophoblast invasion? *Placenta.* 2014;35 Suppl:S57–S63.

69. Huppertz B, Kertschanska S, Demir AY et al. Immunohistochemistry of matrix metalloproteinases (MMP), their substrates, and their inhibitors (TIMP) during trophoblast invasion in the human placenta. *Cell Tissue Res.* 1998;291:133–148.

70. Isaka K, Usuda S, Ito H et al. Expression and activity of matrix metalloproteinase 2 and 9 in human trophoblasts. *Placenta.* 2003;24:53–64.

71. Floridon C, Nielsen O, Hølund B et al. Does plasminogen activator inhibitor-1 (PAI-1) control trophoblast invasion? A study of fetal and maternal tissue in intrauterine, tubal and molar pregnancies. *Placenta.* 2000;21:754–762.

72. Red-Horse K, Zhou Y, Genbacev O et al. Trophoblast differentiation during embryo implantation and formation of the maternal-fetal interface. *J Clin Invest.* 2004;114:744–754.

73. Muttukrishna S, Suri S, Groome N, Jauniaux E. Relationships between TGF-beta proteins and oxygen concentrations inside the first trimester human gestational sac. *PLoS One.* 2008;3:e2302.

74. Schanz A, Red-Horse K, Hess AP et al. Oxygen regulates human cytotrophoblast migration by controlling chemokine and receptor expression. *Placenta.* 2014;35:1089–1094.

75. Oefner CM, Sharkey A, Gardner L et al. Collagen type IV at the fetal-maternal interface. *Placenta.* 2015;36:59–68.

76. Klar M, Michels KB. Cesarean section and placental disorders in subsequent pregnancies—A meta-analysis. *J Perinat Med.* 2014;42:571–583.
77. Kamara M, Henderson JJ, Doherty DA et al. The risk of placenta accreta following primary elective caesarean delivery: A case-control study. *BJOG.* 2013;120:879–886.
78. Flo K, Widnes C, Vårtun Å, Acharya G. Blood flow to the scarred gravid uterus at 22–24 weeks of gestation. *BJOG.* 2014;121:210–215.
79. Ben-Nagi J, Walker A, Jurkovic D et al. Effect of cesarean delivery on the endometrium. *Int J Gynaecol Obstet.* 2009;106:30–34.
80. Khong TY, Robertson WB. Placenta creta and placenta praevia creta. *Placenta.* 1987;8:399–409.
81. Khong TY. The pathology of placenta accreta, a worldwide epidemic. *J Clin Pathol.* 2008;61:1243–1246.
82. Kim KR, Jun SY, Kim JY, Ro JY. Implantation site intermediate trophoblast in placenta cretas. *Mod Pathol.* 2004;17:1483–1490.
83. Hannon T, Innes BA, Lash GE et al. Effects of local decidua on trophoblast invasion and spiral artery remodeling in focal placenta creta—An immunohistochemical study. *Placenta.* 2012;33:998–1004.
84. Stanek J, Drummond Z. Occult placenta accreta: The missing link in the diagnosis of abnormal placentation. *Pediatr Dev Pathol.* 2007;10:266–273.
85. Tseng JJ, Hsu SL, Wen MC et al. Expression of epidermal growth factor receptor and c-erb β-2 oncoprotein in trophoblast populations of placenta accrete. *Am J Obstet Gynecol.* 2004;191:2106–2113.
86. Tseng JJ, Chou MM, Hsieh YT et al. Differential expression of vascular endothelial growth factor, placental growth factor and their receptors in placentae from pregnancies complicated by placenta accreta. *Placenta.* 2006;27:70–78.
87. Tseng JJ, Hsu SL, Ho ES et al. Differential expression of angiopoietin-1, angiopoietin-2 and Tie receptors in placentas from pregnancies complicated by placenta accreta. *Am J Obstet Gynecol.* 2006;194:564–571.
88. McCool RA, Bombard AT, Bartholomew DA, Calhoun BC. Unexplained positive/elevated maternal serum alpha-fetoprotein associated with placenta increta. A case report. *J Reprod Med.* 1992;37:826–828.
89. Thompson O, Otigbah C, Nnochiri A et al. First trimester maternal serum biochemical markers of aneuploidy in pregnancies with abnormally invasive placentation. *BJOG.* 2015;122:1370–1376.
90. Tantbirojn P, Crum CP, Parast MM. Pathophysiology of placenta creta: The role of decidua and extravillous trophoblast. *Placenta.* 2008;29:639–645.
91. Wehrum MJ, Buhimschi IA, Salafia C et al. Accreta complicating complete placenta previa is characterized by reduced systemic levels of vascular endothelial growth factor and by epithelial-to-mesenchymal transition of the invasive trophoblast. *Am J Obstet Gynecol.* 2011;204:411.
92. Achen MG, Gad JM, Stacker SA, Wilks AF. Placenta growth factor and vascular endothelial growth factor are co-expressed during early embryonic development. *Growth Factors.* 1997;15:69–80.
93. McMahon K, Karumanchi SA, Stillman IE et al. Does soluble fms-like tyrosine kinase-1 regulate placental invasion? Insight from the invasive placenta. *Am J Obstet Gynecol.* 2014;210:68.e1–e4.
94. Parra-Herran C, Djordjevic B. Histopathology of placenta creta: Chorionic villi intrusion into myometrial vascular spaces and extravillous trophoblast proliferation are frequent and specific findings with implications on diagnosis and pathogenesis. *Int J Gynecol Pathol.* 2016;35:497–508.
95. El Behery MM, Rasha LE, El Alfy Y. Cell-free placental mRNA in maternal plasma to predict placental invasion in patients with placenta accreta. *Int J Gynaecol Obstet.* 2010;109:30–33.
96. Zhou J, Li J, Yan P et al. Maternal plasma levels of cell-free β-HCG mRNA as a prenatal diagnostic indicator of placenta accrete. *Placenta.* 2014;35:691–695.
97. Cramer SF, Heller D. Placenta accreta and placenta increta: An approach to pathogenesis based on the trophoblastic differentiation pathway. *Pediatr Dev Pathol.* 2016;19:320–333.
98. Jauniaux E, Collins SL, Jurkovic D, Burton GJ. Accreta placentation. A systematic review of prenatal ultrasound imaging and grading of villous invasiveness. *Am J Obstet Gynecol.* 2016;215:712–21.
99. Dannheim K, Shainker SA, Hecht JL. Hysterectomy for placenta accreta; methods for gross and microscopic pathology examination. *Arch Gynecol Obstet.* 2016;293:951–958.
100. Alfirevic Z, Tang A-W, Collins SL, Robson SC, Palacios-Jaraquemadas J; Ad-hoc International AIP Expert group. Pro forma for ultrasound reporting in suspected abnormally invasive placenta (AIP): an international consensus. *Ultrasound Obstet Gynecol.* 2016;47:276–278.

3

Ultrasound Diagnosis of the Morbidly Adherent Placenta

Eliza M. Berkley and Alfred Abuhamad

CONTENTS

Introduction

Morbidly adherent placenta is a novel pathologic entity. It was first described in the 20th century and reported in the 1930s. This suggests that this entity did not exist, or at least was quite rare, before the 1930s.[1] This is probably related to the rare occurrence of cesarean deliveries prior to the 1900s and thus the occurrence of morbidly adherent placentas was uncommon. The diagnosis of morbidly adherent placenta can be made with sonography. In this chapter, we present the ultrasonographic markers of morbidly adherent placenta and discuss ways to optimize its diagnosis by ultrasound.

Definition

The term morbidly adherent placenta implies abnormal implantation of the placenta into the uterine wall. This term has been used to describe placenta accreta, increta, and percreta. Placenta accreta occurs when the placental villi adhere directly to the myometrium, a placenta increta involves placental villi invading into myometrium, and a placenta percreta is defined as placental villi invading through myometrium and into serosa and, sometimes, adjacent organs. About 75% of morbidly adherent placentas are placenta accretas, 18% are placenta incretas, and 7% are placenta percretas.[2] The depth of placental invasion is clinically important as it affects the risk of hemorrhage, injury to other organs, and consequently, management. In this chapter, we use the term placenta accreta interchangeably with morbidly adherent placenta. Placenta accretas can be subdivided into total placenta accreta, partial placenta accreta, or focal placenta accreta based upon the amount of placental tissue that is attached to the myometrium. Pathogenesis of placenta accreta is not clear. There are several theories. The most prominent current theory is abnormal vascularization resulting from the scarring process after uterine surgery with secondary localized hypoxia leading to both defective decidualization and excessive trophoblastic invasion.[3-5]

Clinical Presentation

Most patients with placenta accreta are asymptomatic. Symptoms related to placenta accreta may include vaginal bleeding and cramping. These findings are most common in women with placenta previa, which along with prior cesarean delivery are the strongest risk factors for an accreta.

The overall incidence of placenta accreta is around three per 1000 deliveries and there has been a significant increase in the incidence of placenta accreta over the past several decades.[6,7] The main reason for this increase is the concurrent rise in cesarean section rates. In a large maternal–fetal medicine network study published in 2006, a strong association between placenta previa and placenta accreta was noted, especially in women with prior cesarean section.[8] In this study, the presence of prior cesarean section in a patient significantly increased the risk of placenta accreta, especially in the presence of a placenta previa.[8] It is critical, therefore, to perform an ultrasound assessing for the presence of a placenta previa in patients with prior cesarean sections. Moreover, in women with placenta previa, the risk of accreta increases with increasing numbers of cesarean deliveries.

Accurate prenatal diagnosis of placenta accreta is essential in order to minimize complications and optimize management. Complications of placenta accreta are many and include damage to local organs, postoperative bleeding, amniotic fluid embolism, coagulopathy, transfusion-related complications, acute respiratory distress syndrome, postoperative thromboembolism, infectious morbidities, multisystem organ failure, and maternal death.[9]

Sonographic Findings

Ultrasound is the most commonly used imaging modality for the diagnosis of placenta accreta. As studies evaluate the overall predictive accuracy of ultrasound in detecting placenta accreta, it has become important to evaluate each sonographic marker's contribution to the diagnosis. Many early studies included small sample size and retrospective study designs, which confounded results. Recent studies have reviewed the sensitivity, specificity, and positive and negative predictive values for each marker, and some have proposed scoring or grading systems. We will attempt to review the significance of each sonographic marker and will present an approach to the diagnosis of placenta accreta at various gestations.

Before we describe the sonographic features of placenta accreta, it is important to consider the sonographic approach and its optimization. The authors believe that the diagnosis of placenta accreta should not be performed solely with transabdominal sonogram, unless there is an absolute contraindication to transvaginal ultrasound (very rare). The transvaginal sonographic approach to the evaluation of the placenta allows for higher resolution, which enhances visualization. The presence of an associated placenta previa is thus confirmed, the invasion of cervical tissue by placenta accreta can be clearly noted and the posterior bladder wall, along with the internal aspects of the bladder, can be evaluated. Furthermore, the application of color Doppler in low velocity allows assessment of the extent of placental and lower segment vascularization. Table 3.1 shows the steps for optimization of the ultrasound approach in the evaluation for placenta accreta.

First Trimester Markers

The sonographic findings of placenta accreta in early gestation primarily include a gestational sac (GS) that is implanted in the lower uterine segment (Figure 3.1), a GS that is embedded in a cesarean section scar (Figure 3.2), and the presence of multiple vascular spaces (lacunae) within the placental bed (see

TABLE 3.1

Optimization of the Ultrasound Examination in Placenta Accreta

Use a Combined Transvaginal and Transabdominal Approach
Adjust focal zone(s) to the region of interest.
On transabdominal approach, magnify placenta and scan it in its entirety.
On transvaginal approach, reduce sector width, but ensure posterior bladder wall is in view.
Add color Doppler in low velocity scales and low filters.
Save images and/or movie clips of placenta.

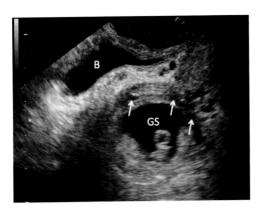

FIGURE 3.1   Sagittal view of the uterus in a low uterine segment implantation of the gestational sac (GS) in a pregnancy with three prior cesarean sections. See the location of the GS in the lower uterine segment posterior to the bladder (B). Note the presence of multiple vascular lacunaes (arrows) within the placenta, representing another sonographic sign of placenta accreta in early gestation. This pregnancy resulted in a placenta percreta.

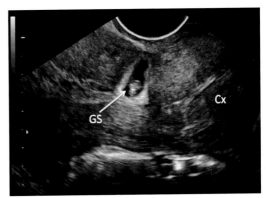

FIGURE 3.2   Sagittal view of the lower uterine segment and the cervix in a cesarean section scar implantation of the GS in a pregnancy with one prior cesarean section. See the location of the GS embedded in the cesarean section scar. Cx: cervix.

Figure 3.1). Ballas defines lower uterine segment implantation as a GS implanted in the lower third of the uterus between 8 and 10 weeks or primarily occupying the lower uterine segment from 10 weeks onward.[10] One must, however, differentiate pregnancies at significant risk for placenta accreta from an ongoing pregnancy loss. With the application of color Doppler, a failing pregnancy can be clearly distinguished as a sac that lacks circumferential blood flow, in addition to a sac that moves when pressure is applied to the anterior surface of the uterus.[11] In a retrospective study evaluating early sonographic appearance of placenta accreta, seven cases of placenta accreta had ultrasound examinations prior to 10 weeks gestation. Six of the seven revealed a low-lying GS near the cervix in patients with prior cesarean section while one sac was implanted near the uterine fundus. In the six cases with lower uterine segment implantations, two had first trimester losses in which dilation and curettage was performed and both ultimately needed hysterectomies for excessive hemorrhage. The four near-term deliveries required three cesarean hysterectomies and one uterine artery embolization after a vaginal delivery with persistent bleeding.[12]

Not all GSs that implant in the lower uterine segment lead to placenta accretas, as subsequent normal pregnancies have been reported. In these instances, a normal thick anterior myometrium superior to the GS and a continuous white line representing the bladder–uterine wall interface is seen on ultrasound.[12] The GS should be contiguous with the endometrial cavity.[11]

In patients with a prior cesarean section, pregnancies implanted in the lower uterine segment carry significant risk for placenta accreta. In these cases, the GS typically implants in or near the cesarean section scar, the anterior myometrium appears thin, and the placental–myometrial and bladder–uterine wall interfaces often appear irregular (see Figure 3.2).[11] The term cesarean scar pregnancy should be differentiated from a low uterine segment implantation as the former implies a GS that is embedded within the cesarean section scar.

Many studies combine cesarean scar pregnancies with pregnancies that implant in the lower uterine segment, near the cesarean section scar.[9] A true cesarean scar pregnancy should be implanted within the myometrium, surrounded on all sides by myometrium, and be separate from the endometrium (see Figure 3.2). Color Doppler in a low-velocity scale demonstrates surrounding vascularity of placental tissue (Figure 3.3). If untreated, cesarean section scar implantation may lead to significant abnormalities in the placenta with placenta accreta, percreta, and increta. Although it may be useful to distinguish between true scar pregnancies and lower uterine segment implantations adjacent to or involving the scar, both carry considerable risk for placenta accreta and excessive hemorrhage and the approach to treatment of both conditions is similar.

Early diagnosis of these pregnancies may improve prognosis and decrease the need for hysterectomy.[13] There are typically three treatment modalities: surgical treatment (abdominal or transvaginal), direct injection of methotrexate (or potassium chloride) into the GS, or expectant management. A study evaluating management and outcomes of 18 cases of pregnancies implanted into the cesarean section scar, all diagnosed in the first trimester, showed benefit of early diagnosis and intervention.[13] Similar to other studies, a low-lying GS near the cervix was noted on ultrasound with a thin or absent anterior myometrium and bulging through the uterine wall with close proximity to the bladder. Of note, 44% of these cases ended in spontaneous first trimester pregnancy loss but still required obstetric management for resolution. Eight of the 18 cases initially had ultrasound-guided suction dilation and curettage. All of these were successful and needed no further surgical treatment. Seven cases received medical treatment with methotrexate or methotrexate and potassium chloride directly injected into the GS, with an overall success rate of 71%. Two of these cases subsequently underwent a dilation and curettage and one of them also required uterine artery embolization. Both of these cases also received transfusions for estimated blood losses of over 1000 mL. Resolution of human chorionic gonadotropin (HCG) levels took 6–10 weeks. Expectant management was successful in only one of three cases.[13] The maternal outcome of cesarean section scar pregnancy treated in the first trimester seems to be better than placenta accreta treated later in gestation. As such, the authors currently recommend treatment of cesarean scar implantation with direct GS injection of methotrexate under ultrasound guidance.

Of note, over the last 5 years, several articles have discussed the use of balloon catheters placed in the cervical canal or uterine cavity for treatment of hemorrhage secondary to cervical or cesarean scar pregnancies.[14,15] A recent retrospective study of 18 such cases discussed the use of a Foley balloon placed into the uterus under transvaginal ultrasound guidance and reported that it was easy to perform, well tolerated by the patients, decreased complications from severe bleeding, and decreased surgical

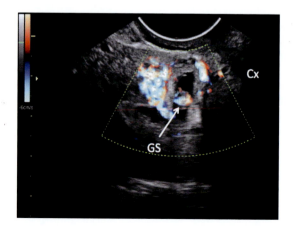

FIGURE 3.3 Color Doppler of a sagittal view of the lower uterine segment and the cervix in a cesarean section scar implantation of the GS in a pregnancy with one prior cesarean section (same as in Figure 3.2). Note the presence of vascularity on color Doppler surrounding the GS. Cx: cervix.

intervention. In eight subjects, the Foley balloon was placed immediately after methotrexate injection, in another eight it was placed days later following suction aspiration, and two had Foley catheter placement several days later after the sudden onset of severe hemorrhage. In all but one case the desired tamponade effect was achieved and follow-up ultrasound studies revealed regression of vascularization.[14] In light of this data, we suggest using a balloon catheter as a prophylactic method or adjuvant treatment in the management of cervical pregnancies or cesarean scar pregnancies. More longitudinal studies are required before we can recommend use of balloon compression as a primary treatment modality for cesarean scar gestation.

The third marker of placenta accreta in the first trimester is the presence of anechoic areas within the placenta with or without documented blood flow on color Doppler (see Figure 3.1).[10,16–19] These anechoic areas have been described as vascular spaces, lacunae, or lakes. Most commonly called placental lacunae, they were first described as a possible marker for placenta accreta by Kerr de Mendonca in 1988. Since that time, multiple case reports of these hypoechoic vascular spaces noted on ultrasound at less than 12 weeks have linked them to the early diagnosis of placenta accreta. If the pregnancy progresses these lacunae become more prominent in the second and third trimester. Three examples of irregularly shaped placental lacunae diagnosed at 8th, 9th, and 12th weeks were reported in women presenting with vaginal bleeding and suspicion for abnormal placentation.[16,18,19] Two resulted in a hysterectomy secondary to hemorrhage as early as 15 weeks and placenta accreta was confirmed. In the third case, the patient elected termination and the uterus was preserved. A retrospective study by Ballas et al. further confirms lacunae as a first trimester marker for placenta accreta. They reported on 10 cases of placenta accreta with first trimester ultrasounds and noted that anechoic placental areas were present in 8 of 10 (80%).[10]

Second and Third Trimester Markers

Multiple markers have been used to diagnose placenta accreta in the second and third trimesters of pregnancy. Table 3.2 lists common second and third trimester sonographic markers described in association with placental accreta.

Multiple Vascular Lacunae

Multiple vascular lacunae within the placenta in the second and third trimester of pregnancy (Figure 3.4) have been correlated with high sensitivity and low false-positive rate for placenta accreta.[20] It is important that lacunae are differentiated from placental lakes. Lacunae appear deeper in the placenta, typically have an irregular border, and when color Doppler is applied have turbulent flow with high velocity and low impedance (Figure 3.5).[20] Lacunae have been reported as early as 8 weeks and are commonly seen as sonographic markers for placenta accreta and percreta in the second and third trimester. Placental lacunae in the second trimester with turbulent blood flow on Doppler ultrasonography are associated with placenta accreta. Some studies report lacunae to have the highest sensitivity and positive predictive value when compared to other markers for placenta accreta.[20] However, the predictive value of lacunae varies by study with a range of sensitivity between 73% and 100% and negative predictive value of

TABLE 3.2

Second and Third Trimester Sonographic Markers of Placental Accreta

Multiple Vascular Lacunae
Loss of the normal hypoechoic retroplacental zone
Abnormality of the uterine serosa–bladder interface
Thinning of the retroplacental myometrium
Bulging of the lower uterine segment
Increased placental vascularity on color Doppler

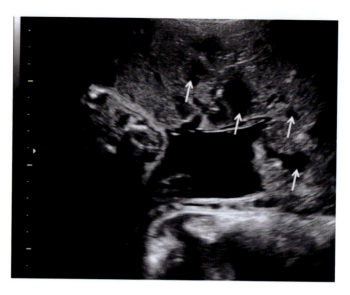

FIGURE 3.4 Sagittal view of the lower uterine segment in grayscale ultrasound in a patient with placenta accreta. Note the presence of multiple anechoic spaces within the placenta, corresponding to placental lacunaes (arrows). Some studies have correlated the presence of four or more placental lacunaes with a high prevalence of placenta accreta (see text for details).

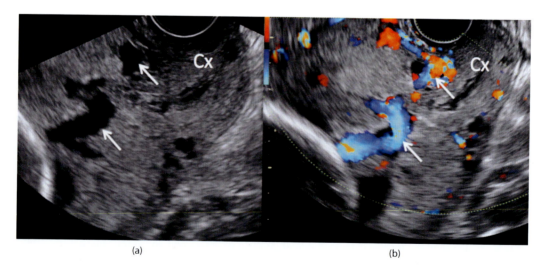

(a)   (b)

FIGURE 3.5 Sagittal view of the lower uterine segment and cervix in grayscale (a) and color Doppler (b) ultrasound in a patient with placenta accreta. Note the presence of multiple anechoic spaces within the placenta in (a), corresponding to placental lacunaes (arrows). Color Doppler in (b) shows vascular flow within the lacunaes. Cx: cervix.

88%–100%.[20] There is an agreement, however, that the greater the number of lacunae, the higher the risk for placenta accreta and even percreta. Multiple vascular lacunae within the placenta, or a Swiss-cheese appearance (see Figure 3.4), is one of the most important sonographic findings of placenta accreta in the second and third trimester. The pathogenesis of this finding is probably related to placental tissue alterations resulting from long-term exposure to pulsatile blood flow.[21,22] When multiple lacunae are seen, especially four or more, the association with placenta accreta has been reported at 100% in some studies.[23,24] This marker also has been reported to have a low false-positive rate, but this may not be true in the general population. Lacunaes are common in normal placentas, especially when a placenta previa is not present. It should also be noted that placenta accretas have been reported in the absence of multiple vascular lacunae.[25]

Loss of the Hypoechoic Retroplacental Zone

Loss of the normal hypoechoic (clear) retroplacental zone (Figure 3.6), also referred to as loss of the clear space between the placenta and the uterus, is another marker for placenta accreta.[26,27] This sonographic finding has been reported to have a detection rate of about 93%, with a sensitivity of 52% and a specificity of 57%. The false positive rate, however, has been in the range of 21% or higher. This marker should not be used alone as it is angle dependent and can be found (absent clear zone) in normal anterior placentas.[25–28] The strength of this ultrasound marker is in its negative predictive value, which ranges from 96% to 100%. The presence of a hypoechoic retroplacental clear space that extends the length of the placenta (Figure 3.7) makes the placenta accreta unlikely.[23,29]

Uterine Serosa–Posterior Bladder Wall Interface

Multiple studies also reported that abnormalities of the uterine serosa–bladder interface are predictive of placenta accreta. This includes interruption of the line, thickening of the line, irregularity of the line, or increase vascularity on color Doppler (Figures 3.8 and 3.9).[30,31] The normal uterine

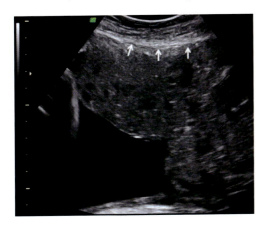

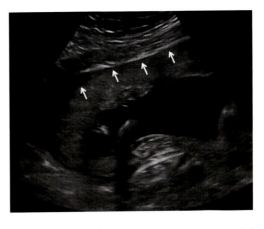

FIGURE 3.6 Transabdominal ultrasound in gray scale in a pregnancy with an anterior placental accreta. Note the absence of the hypoechoic zone (arrows) between the placenta and the uterine wall. Compare with a normal placenta in Figure 3.7.

FIGURE 3.7 Transabdominal ultrasound in gray scale in a pregnancy with an anterior-fundal normal placenta. Note the normal appearance of the retroplacental hypoechoic zone (arrows) between the placenta and the uterine wall. Compare with a placenta accreta in Figure 3.6.

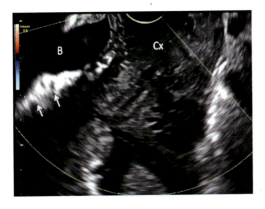

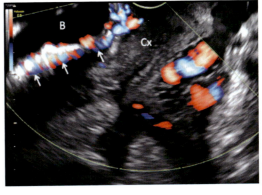

FIGURE 3.8 Transvaginal ultrasound of a sagittal view of the lower uterine segment in a pregnancy with a placenta previa and accreta. Note the presence of increased echogenicity and thickening of the posterior bladder wall (arrows). B: bladder, Cx: cervix.

FIGURE 3.9 Transvaginal ultrasound of a sagittal view of the lower uterine segment in color Doppler in a pregnancy with a placenta previa and accreta (same as in Figure 3.8). Note the presence of increased vascularity of the posterior bladder wall–lower uterine segment interface (arrows). B: bladder, Cx: cervix.

serosa–bladder interface appears as a smooth line with no irregularities or increased vascularity on sagittal imaging (Figure 3.10). Abnormalities of this uterine serosa–bladder interface line include thickening irregularities, increased vascularities, such as varicosities and bulging of the placenta into the posterior wall of the bladder. This finding may be seen as early as the first trimester but is more commonly noted in the second and third trimesters.[17] Initially, this marker was believed to be highly specific, near 100%, but not very sensitive.[30,31] It was helpful in cases of placenta percreta but less diagnostic when there was no bladder invasion. However, when color Doppler is applied to the uterine–bladder interface and a transvaginal approach is used, the sensitivity and specificity for all types of morbidly adherent placenta is high. In fact, a recent meta-analysis reported that irregularity of this interface was the most specific marker for invasive placentation (99.75 CI; 99.5%–99.9%).[32] The contribution of color Doppler and a transvaginal approach improves sensitivity from 70% to 90%.[29] Under these conditions, specificity reaches 99% and the positive and negative predictive values are 96% and 92%, respectively.[29]

Retroplacental Myometrial Thickness

Another ultrasound finding characteristic for placenta accreta is a retroplacental myometrial thickness less than 1 mm.[33,34] This is difficult to assess since the lower uterine segment myometrium thins in normal pregnancy as term is approached. In patients with at least one prior cesarean section, the median myometrial thickness of the lower uterine segment in the third trimester is 2.4 mm.[35] Thinning of the myometrium in the upper uterine segment should always be of concern. Previous studies on this marker have reported a range of sensitivity between 22% and 100% and specificity between 100% and 72%.[33,34] Given this variation, it is important to standardize the gestational age and sonographic approach for this marker.

Increased Placental Vascularity on Color Doppler

Color Doppler may be used as an adjunct to two-dimensional (2D) ultrasound in the diagnosis of placenta accreta. Color Doppler helps differentiate the normal subplacental venous complex with nonpulsatile low-velocity venous blood flow waveforms from the presence of markedly dilated peripheral subplacental vascular channels with pulsatile venous-type flow, suggestive of a morbidly adherent placenta (Figure 3.11). These vascular channels are often located directly over the cervix (see Figure 3.11). In addition, the observation of bridging vessels linking the placenta and bladder with high diastolic arterial blood flow is also suggestive for invasion.[30,36] Two small-scale studies reported the sensitivity of

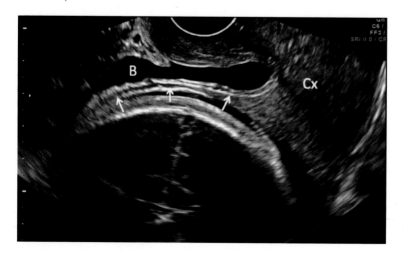

FIGURE 3.10 Transvaginal ultrasound of a sagittal view of the lower uterine segment in gray scale in a normal pregnancy. Note the thin, uniform shape of the posterior bladder wall–lower uterine segment interface (arrows). B: bladder, Cx: cervix.

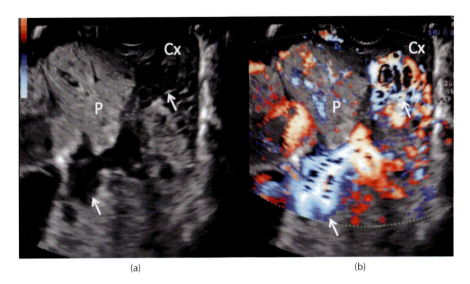

FIGURE 3.11 Sagittal view of the lower uterine segment and cervix in grayscale (a) and color Doppler (b) ultrasound in a patient with placenta previa and accreta. Note the presence of multiple anechoic spaces within the placenta in (a), corresponding to placental lacunaes (arrows). Color Doppler in (b) shows extensive vascular flow within the lacunaes. Cx: cervix, P: placenta.

color Doppler imaging for the diagnosis of invasive placenta between 86% and 100% and the specificity between 94% and 92%.[37,38]

Placental Bulge

Other proposed ultrasound markers for morbidly adherent placenta include the presence of a placental bulge or focal exophytic mass. Deviation of the uterine serosa creating an abnormal placental shape or bulge of placental tissue into neighboring structures, most commonly the bladder, can occasionally be seen. While this indicates a possible placenta accreta it is not necessarily suggestive for percreta. Even more concerning is disruption of the uterine serosa with placental extension suggestive of an exophytic mass.[30,39]

Studies have also evaluated the role of three-dimensional (3D) ultrasound in the prediction of placenta accreta. The application of 3D ultrasound in vascular mode has shown promise as it allows for a semi-quantitative assessment of placental vasculature.[40,41] Drawbacks exist, however, for the application of 3D ultrasound in screening for placenta accreta. This technology currently is not well standardized and requires significant operator expertise for volume acquisition and manipulation. Prospective studies are therefore needed before the routine application of 3D ultrasound in screening and diagnosis of placenta accreta.

Diagnostic Accuracy of Ultrasound

In 2013, a systematic review and meta-analysis of the prenatal identification of invasive placentation assessed the diagnostic accuracy of the following individual sonographic markers: placental lacunae, loss of the hypoechoic space between the placenta and the myometrium, abnormalities at the uterus–bladder interface, and color Doppler abnormalities. They report diagnostic accuracy of 0.89, 0.88, 0.93, and 0.95, respectively. Color Doppler had the best predictive accuracy. Of note, many of the earlier studies did not employ color Doppler for the diagnosis of placenta accreta. It is likely that its inclusion would improve the sensitivity and specificity of ultrasound in the diagnosis of invasive placentation.[32]

Overall, grayscale ultrasonography appears to be an excellent tool for the prenatal diagnosis of placenta accreta in women at risk. Its sensitivity has been reported in the range of 77%–87%, with a specificity of 96%–98%, a positive predictive value of 65%–93%, and a negative predictive value of 98%.[42] A meta-analysis in 2013 reported a pooled sensitivity of 83%.[43]

In contrast, another recent study suggested that the true predictive power of ultrasound to diagnose placenta accreta is actually less than previously reported.[32] The authors report that initial studies assessing the accuracy of ultrasound prediction of placenta accreta may be biased from the inclusion of single expert observations, known suspicion for accreta, and knowledge of risk factors. In addition, small sample sizes, retrospective designs, and wide variability in the definition and inclusion criteria led to inconsistency in performance and skewed sensitivity.[32] When investigators are blinded to clinical history and multiple experienced providers review the same ultrasound images, the accuracy of diagnosing placenta accreta declines. The sensitivity, specificity, positive and negative predictive values, and accuracy drop to 54%, 88%, 82%, 65%, and 65%, respectively, according to the largest prospective study of accreta patients to date.[44] The true sensitivity and specificity likely lie somewhere in between as practitioners are typically aware of patient risk factors and history and can use real-time sonographic imaging and 3D techniques.

In addition to the number and variation of sonographic markers used in the diagnosis of placenta accreta, recent studies underscore a need to standardize the technique for evaluating each proposed marker. For example, abnormality of the uterine serosa–bladder interface can be assessed with transabdominal or transvaginal ultrasound and with an empty or full bladder. The transvaginal approach with a partially full bladder appears to improve sensitivity and specificity of this marker to 70% and 99%, respectively.[29] Further support for standardization of the diagnosis of each marker and the techniques used for assessment are provided by an evaluation of interobserver variability in the diagnosis of placenta accreta. This study reported wide variability with a kappa value ranging from 0.32 to 0.74. In order to decrease variability and improve the ultrasound diagnosis of placenta accreta it is important to define and standardize the diagnosis of each sonographic marker for placenta accreta.[44]

In fact, an international group of experts called the European Working Group on Abnormally Invasive Placenta (AIP) was recently assembled to produce a consensus proposal for standardization of ultrasound descriptions used to define each marker/sign. The goal was to develop a form for standard ultrasound evaluation for invasive placentation (Table 3.3). If adopted by clinicians, sonographers, and researchers it would improve communication, make evaluation more consistent with a systematic approach, and allow true assessment of the diagnostic performance of each ultrasound marker or combination of markers. The ultimate goal is to determine the true likelihood of morbidly adherent placenta or at least stratify a patient's risk into low, intermediate, or high and thus reduce maternal morbidity and perinatal complications.[45] The authors agree that this represents an important first step toward standardization of markers of placenta accreta. However, some of the proposed definitions do not allow for consistency, such as lack of clear definition for placental lacuna.

Although studies vary on the exact sensitivity and positive predictive value of ultrasound in the diagnosis of placenta accreta, almost all agree that ultrasound should be the primary imaging modality and should be used exclusively in the great majority of cases.[46] Magnetic resonance imaging (MRI) is the other imaging modality that is commonly used. The overall reported sensitivity of the MRI is 80%–85% with a specificity of 65%–100%,[26] which is comparable to ultrasound. However, studies are smaller and more prone to bias than those conducted using ultrasound. Few studies comparing the two have been done and all are small and lack statistical power. MRI may be complementary to ultrasound in cases where the placenta is posterior or located laterally.[47] It is important to know that when an MRI was used in conjunction with ultrasound in assessing patients for the diagnosis of placenta accreta, MRI was rarely helpful in changing surgical management. One exception may lie in MRI's ability to assess the degree/depth of invasion of the placenta and discerning placenta percreta from accreta.[48]

TABLE 3.3

Proposed Standardized Ultrasound Markers for the Diagnosis of Placenta Accreta

US Finding	EW-AIP Suggested Standardized Definition
2D grayscale	
Loss of "clear zone" (Figure 3.1)	Loss, or irregularity, of hypoechoic plane in myometrium underneath placental bed ("clear zone")
Abnormal placental lacunae (Figure 3.2)	Presence of numerous lacunae including some that are large and irregular (Finberg Grade 3), often containing turbulent flow visible on grayscale imaging
Bladder wall interruption (Figure 3.3)	Loss or interruption of bright bladder wall (hyperechoic band or "line" between uterine serosa and bladder lumen)
Myometrial thinning (Figure 3.4)	Thinning of myometrium overlying placenta to <1 mm or undetectable
Placental bulge (Figure 3.5)	Deviation of uterine serosa away from expected plane, caused by abnormal bulge of placental tissue into neighboring organ, typically bladder; uterine serosa appears intact but outline shape is distorted
Focal exophytic mass (Figure 3.6)	Placental tissue seen breaking through uterine serosa and extending beyond it; most often seen inside filled urinary bladder
2D color Doppler	
Uterovesical hypervascularity (Figure 3.7)	Striking amount of color Doppler signal seen between myometrium and posterior wall of bladder; this sign probably indicates numerous, closely packed, tortuous vessels in that region (demonstrating multidirectional flow and aliasing artifact)
Subplacental hypervascularity (Figure 3.8)	Striking amount of color Doppler signal seen in placental bed; this sign probably indicates numerous, closely packed, tortuous vessels in that region (demonstrating multidirectional flow and aliasing artifact)
Bridging vessels (Figure 3.9)	Vessels appearing to extend from placenta, across myometrium and beyond serosa into bladder or other organs; often running perpendicular to myometrium
Placental lacunae feeder vessels (Figure 3.10)	Vessels with high-velocity blood flow leading from myometrium into placental lacunae, causing turbulence upon entry
3D ultrasound ± power Doppler	
Intraplacental hypervascularity (Figure 3.11)	Complex, irregular arrangement of numerous placental vessels, exhibiting tortuous courses and varying calibers
Placental bulge	(As in 2D)
Focal exophytic mass	(As in 2D)
Uterovesical hypervascularity	(As in 2D)
Bridging vessels	(As in 2D)

Source: Collins S et al., *Ultrasound Obstet Gynecol,* 47, 271–275, 2016. With permission.

Conclusion

Placenta accreta is a major complication of pregnancy with substantial maternal morbidity and mortality. Prenatal diagnosis of placenta accreta minimizes pregnancy complications as it allows for a multidisciplinary approach to care and planning for delivery. Undoubtedly, ultrasound markers of placenta accreta play a significant role in prenatal diagnosis. The presence of multiple vascular placental lacunae, increased placental vascularity, and/or posterior bladder wall abnormalities appear to play a critical role in ultrasound diagnosis. It is important to note, however, that the presence of prior cesarean deliveries in association with a placenta previa substantially increases the risk for an accreta.

The extent that each ultrasound marker contributes to the diagnosis is currently unclear as available data are mostly derived from retrospective studies with confounding variables. Standardization of definitions of placental markers and prospective studies are needed in order to further refine and evaluate the prenatal diagnosis of placenta accreta by ultrasound. National registries are being developed as initial steps toward that goal. In the meantime, the authors recommend that physicians and sonographers involved in prenatal care should familiarize themselves with risk factors and ultrasound markers of placenta accreta. Finally, comprehensive evaluation of the placenta by the transvaginal approach is recommended in women at risk for placenta accreta and a high level of suspicion should be employed when ultrasound markers are noted in this setting.

REFERENCES

1. Hertig IC. A study of placenta accreta. *J Surg Gynecol Obstet.* 1937;64:178–200.
2. Miller D, Chollet JA, Goodwin TM. Clinical risk factors for placenta previa-placenta accreta. *Am J Obstet Gynecol.* 1997;177(1):210–214.
3. Wehrum MJ, Buhimschi IA, Salafia C et al. Accreta complicating complete placenta previa is characterized by reduced systemic levels of vascular endothelial growth factor and by epithelial-to-mesenchymal transition of the invasive trophoblast. *Am J Obstet Gynecol.* 2011;204(5):e1–e411.
4. Tantbirojn P, Crum CP, Parast MM. Pathophysiology of placenta accreta: The roll of deciduas and extravillous trophoblast. *Placenta.* 2008;29(7):639–645.
5. Strickland S, Richards WG. Invasion of the trophoblast. *Cell.* 1992;71:355–357.
6. Belfort MA. Placenta accreta. *Am J Obstet Gynecol.* 2010;203(5):430–439.
7. Hull AD, Resnik R. Placenta accreta and postpartum hemorrhage. *Clin Obstet Gynecol.* 2010;53(1):228–236.
8. Silver RM, Landon MB, Rouse DJ et al. Maternal morbidity associated with multiple repeat cesarean deliveries. *Obstet Gynecol.* 2006;107(6):1226–1232.
9. O'Brien JM, Barton JR, Donaldson ES. The management of placenta percreta: Conservative and operative strategies. *Am J Obstet Gynecol.* 1996;175(6):1632–1638.
10. Ballas J, Pretorius D, Hull AD, Resnik R, Ramos AG. Identifying sonographic markers for placenta accreta in the first trimester. *Am J Obstet Gynecol.* 2012;31:1835–1841.
11. Comstock CH, Bronsteen RA. The antenatal diagnosis of placenta accreta. *BJOG.* 2014;121:171–182.
12. Comstock CH, Wesley L, Vettraino IM, Bronsteen RA. The early sonographic appearance of placenta accreta. *J Ultrasound Med.* 2003;22(1):19–23.
13. Jurkovic D, Hillaby K, Woelfer B, Lawrence A, Salim R, Elson CJ. First-trimester diagnosis and management of pregnancies implanted into the lower uterine segment cesarean section scar. *Ultrasound Obstet Gynecol.* 2003;21:220–227.
14. Timor-Tritsch IE, Cali G, Monteagudo A et al. Foley balloon catheter to prevent or manage bleeding during treatment for cervical and cesarean scar pregnancy. *Ultrasound Obstet Gynecol.* 2015;46:118–123.
15. Jiang T, Liu G, Huang L, Ma H, Zhang S. Methotrexate therapy followed by suction curettage followed by Foley tamponade for cesarean scar pregnancy. *Eur J Obstet Gynecol.* 2011;156(2):209–211.
16. Chen YJ, Wang PH, Liu WM, Lai CR, Shu LP, Hung JH. Placenta accreta diagnosed at 9 weeks' gestation. *Ultrasound Obstet Gynecol.* 2002;19:620–622.
17. Wong HS, Zuccollo J, Tait J, Pringle KC. Placenta accreta in the first trimester of pregnancy: Sonographic findings. *J Clin Ultrasound* 2007;37:100–102.
18. Yang JI, Kim HY, Kim HS, Ryu HS. Diagnosis in the first trimester of placenta accreta with previous cesarean section. *Ultrasound Obstet Gynecol.* 2009;34:116–118.
19. Shih JC, Cheng WF, Shyu MK, Lee CN, Hsieh FJ. Power Doppler evidence of placenta accreta appearing in the first trimester. *Ultrasound Obstet Gynecol.* 2002;19:623–625.
20. Comstock CH, Love JJ, Bronsteen RA, Lee W, Vettraino IM, Huang RR. Sonographic detection of placenta accreta in the second and third trimesters of pregnancy. *Am J Obstet Gynecol.* 2004;190(4):1135–1140.
21. Hull AD, Salerno CC, Saenz CC, Pretorius DH. Three-dimensional ultrasonography and diagnosis of placenta percreta with bladder involvement. *J Ultrasound Med.* 1999;18(12):853–856.
22. Baughman WC, Corteville JE, Shah RR. Placenta accreta: Spectrum of US and MR imaging findings. *Radiographics.* 2008;28(7):1905–1916.

23. Wong HS, Cheung YK, Zuccollo J, Tait J, Pringle JC. Evaluation of sonographic diagnostic criteria for placenta accreta. *J Clin Ultrasound.* 2008;36(9):551–559.

24. Yang JI, Lim YK, Kim HS, Chang KH, Lee JP, Ryu HS. Sonographic findings of placental lacunae and the prediction of adherent placenta in women with placenta previa totalis and prior cesarean section. *Ultrasound Obstet Gynecol.* 2006;28:178–182.

25. Finberg HJ, Williams JW. Placenta accreta: Prospective sonographic diagnosis in patients with placenta previa and prior cesarean section. *J Ultrasound Med.* 1992;11(7):333–343.

26. Gielchinsky Y, Mankuta D, Rojansky N, Laufer N, Gielchinsky I, Ezra Y. Perinatal outcome of pregnancies complicated by placenta accreta. *Obstet Gynecol.* 2004;104(3):527–530.

27. Hudon L, Belfort MA, Broome DR. Diagnosis and management of placenta percreta: A review. *Obstet Gynecol Surv.* 1998;53(8):509–517.

28. Royal College of Obstetricians and Gynaecologists (RCOG). Placenta praevia, placenta praevia accreta and vasa praevia: Diagnosis and management. *Royal College of Obstetricians and Gynaecologists (RCOG)* 2011;26. (Green-top guideline; no. 27.)

29. Cali G, Giambanco L, Puccio G, Forlani F. Morbidly adherent placenta: Evaluation of ultrasound diagnostic criteria and differentiation of placenta accreta from percreta. *Ultrasound Obstet Gynecol.* 2013;41:406–412.

30. Comstock CH. Antenatal diagnosis of placenta accreta: A review. *Ultrasound Obstet Gynecol.* 2005;26(1):89–96.

31. Warshak CR, Eskander R, Hull AD et al. Accuracy of ultrasonography and magnetic resonance imaging in the diagnosis of placenta accreta. *Obstet Gynecol.* 2006;108(3):573–581.

32. D'Antonio F, Iacovella C, Bhide A. Prenatal identification of invasive placentation using ultrasound: Systematic review and meta-analysis. *Ultrasound Obstet Gynecol.* 2013;42:509–517.

33. Twickler DM, Lucas MJ, Balis AB et al. Color flow mapping for myometrial invasion in women with a prior cesarean delivery. *J Matern Fetal Neonatal Med.* 2000;9:330–335.

34. Wong HS, Cheung YK, Strand L et al. Specific sonographic features of placenta accreta: Tissue interface disruption on gray-scale imaging and evidence of vessels crossing interface-disruption sites on Doppler imaging. *Ultrasound Obstet Gynecol.* 2007;29:239–241.

35. Rac MWF, Dasche JS, Wells E, Moschos E, McIntire DD, Twickler DM. Ultrasound predictors of placental invasion: The placenta accreta index. *Am J Obstet Gynecol.* 2015;212(3):343.e1–e7.

36. Chou MM, Ho ES, Lee YH. Prenatal diagnosis of placenta previa accreta by transabdominal color doppler ultrasound. *Ultrasound Obstet Gynecol.* 2000;15(1):28–35.

37. Lerner JP, Deane S, Timor-Tritsch IE. Characterization of placenta accreta using transvaginal sonography and color Doppler imaging. *Ultrasound Obstet Gynecol.* 1995;5:198–201.

38. Levine D, Hulka CA, Ludmir J, Li W, Edelman RR. Placenta accreta: Evaluation with color Doppler US, power Doppler US, and MR imaging. *Radiology.* 1997;205:773–776.

39. Kirkinen P, Helin-Martikainen H, Vanninen R, Partanen K. Placenta accreta: Imaging by gray-scale and contract-enhanced color Doppler sonography and magnetic resonance imaging. *J Clin Ultrasound.* 1998;26:90–94.

40. Collins S, Gordon S, Adbula A et al. Three-dimensional power Doppler ultrasonography for diagnosing abnormally invasive placenta and quantifying the risk. *Obstet Gynecol.* 2015;126(3):645–665.

41. Shih J, Jaraquemada J, Su Y et al. Role of three-dimensional power Doppler in the antenatal diagnosis of placenta accreta: Comparison with gray-scale and color Doppler techniques. *Ultrasound Obstet Gynecol.* 2009;33:193–203.

42. American College of Obstetricians and Gynecologists (ACOG). Placenta accreta. (Committee opinion; no. 529). *Obstet Gynecol.* 2012;120(1):207–211.

43. Meng X, Xie L, Song W. Comparing the diagnostic value of ultrasound and magnetic resonance imaging for placenta accreta: A systematic review and meta-analysis. *Ultrasound Med Biol.* 2013;39:1958–1965.

44. Bowman ZS, Eller AG, Kennedy AM et al. Interobserver variability of sonography for prediction of placenta accreta. *J Clin Ultrasound.* 2014;33:2153–2158.

45. Collins SL, Ashcroft A, Braun T et al. On behalf of the European working group on abnormally invasive placenta. Proposal for standardized descriptors of abnormally invasive placenta (EW-AIP). *Ultrasound Obstet Gynecol.* 2016;47:271–275.

46. Esakoff TF, Sparks TN, Kaimal AJ et al. Diagnosis and morbidity of placenta accrete. *Ultrasound Obstet Gynecol.* 2011;37:324–327.

47. Rezk MA, Shawky M. Grey-scale and colour Doppler ultrasound versus magnetic resonance imaging for the prenatal diagnosis of placenta accreta. *J Matern Fetal Neonatal Med.* 2014;29: e1–e4.

48. D'Antonio F, Iacovella C, Palacios-Jaraquemada J, Bruno CH, Manzolis L, Bhide A. Prenatal identification of invasive placentation using magnetic resonance imaging: Systematic review and meta-analysis. *Ultrasound Obstet Gynecol.* 2014;44:8–16.

4

MRI Diagnosis of Accreta

Andrew D. Hull and Michele A. Brown

CONTENTS

Introduction

There is no doubt that ultrasound is the principal imaging tool for the detection and evaluation of placenta accreta as described elsewhere in this volume. Magnetic resonance imaging (MRI) was first used in pregnancy soon after it was developed, and those early imaging attempts paid particular attention to the placenta.[1-3] At the time, availability of probes for endovaginal ultrasound was limited and researchers and clinicians sought other modalities to evaluate placental location, typically to diagnose placenta previa. Without diagnostic imaging, women with a suspected placenta previa in the late third trimester underwent vaginal examination in an operating room under a "double set-up" prepared for cesarean section. If placenta previa was present, delivery by cesarean section was immediately performed; if not, labor was induced. MRI was an effective tool for placental localization,[4] but was never widely adopted as endovaginal probes became readily available. Later investigators and clinicians turned their attention to MRI as a tool for diagnosis and evaluation of accreta, often with mixed results. In contemporary practice, MRI has a role in the armamentarium of tools used in the diagnosis and management of placenta accreta although its precise application remains controversial.

MRI Technique

Obstetric MRI has evolved over the years with different techniques being proposed and adopted depending on the type of investigation being performed.[5-7] Fetal MRI uses protocols that vary according to the anatomic area of interest and must be modified to reduce movement artifact and allow evaluation of small details of fetal anatomy. Protocols used in placental evaluation have shown a similar pattern of evolution. Although differences exist between individual centers and clinicians, the approach for most studies has become relatively uniform.

At our institution, MR exams are performed using a 1.5-Tesla MRI system with a phased-array torso coil. Patients are imaged without sedation and usually fast for 4 hours prior to imaging because an empty GI tract produces better images. Patients are positioned supine or decubitus based on patient comfort and gestational age. Initial pulse sequences rely on the ultrafast T2-weighted single-shot fast spin echo (SSFSE/HASTE), T2/T1-weighted balanced steady-state free precession (FISP/FIESTA), and T1-weighted gradient spin echo images. Sequences are acquired in at least two orthogonal planes over the region of interest, most commonly the lower uterine segment. High-resolution T2-weighted echo train and spin echo may be helpful when focused upon areas of particularly high suspicion. Gadolinium-based contrast is administered intravenously only if unenhanced images are indeterminate to confirm the diagnosis and assess depth of invasion if the gestational age is 28 weeks or greater. One-half dose of MultiHance® (gadobenate dimeglumine, Bracco Diagnostics Inc., Singen, Germany) is typically sufficient. Dynamic sequences are acquired using two-dimensional (2D) gradient echo, MR angiographic sequences, or modified MR angiographic sequences that speed acquisition time (e.g., time-resolved imaging of contrast kineticS [TRICKS]) to eliminate the need for timing. All patients provide informed consent prior to the exams for both MRI and intravenous contrast administration. A radiologist monitors all studies in order to adequately evaluate the area of interest.

MRI and Safety in Pregnancy

MRI is generally considered to be safe in pregnancy. It does not use ionizing radiation, appears to have no risk of teratogenicity, and does not require special restrictions or precautions.[8,9] There are no published studies documenting harm in human or animal use.[10] Theoretical safety concerns have been raised regarding the use of higher strength magnetic fields (3-Tesla MRI), although no data exist to support evidence of harm.[11] Pregnant patients may require left lateral positioning to reduce caval compression during scanning.

MRI provides good differentiation between tissues without the use of contrast. However, the use of contrast has been advocated in some settings including the evaluation of placenta accreta. There are no data supporting the use or safety of super paramagnetic iron oxide particles in pregnancy and only gadolinium-based contrast should be used. However, the use of gadolinium in pregnancy is controversial.[9,11,12] Gadolinium has not been shown to be teratogenic or mutagenic in animal studies[13] and did not have adverse fetal or newborn effects when used in the first trimester in pregnant women.[14] Free gadolinium is toxic and should only be administered in chelated form; the stability of available compounds varies and it has been suggested that only the most stable compounds be used in pregnancy.[15] Gadolinium crosses the placenta to enter the fetal circulation, is excreted into fetal urine, swallowed as amniotic fluid, is recirculated, and can pass via the placenta to the maternal circulation for final excretion. Concerns have been raised regarding a potential risk of nephrogenic systemic fibrosis (NSF) in neonates exposed to gadolinium in utero because of relatively low fetal and newborn glomerular filtration rate (GFR).[16] An elegant recent study in nonhuman pregnant primates examined the persistence of gadolinium in amniotic fluid and accumulation of gadolinium in fetal tissues following a clinically relevant dose of contrast.[17] The authors found minimal residual gadolinium in amniotic fluid 21 hours after injection and evidence of continuing excretion. Despite these reassuring findings, current recommendations are to restrict gadolinium use to the most stable agents and to use contrast only when benefits clearly outweigh potential risk.[9,15] We believe it is a reasonable option in the third trimester.

MRI and Normal Placenta

It is essential that one can identify the appearance of normal placenta before attempting to evaluate abnormal placentation.[18,19] It also is important to consider the changes that occur in placental anatomy over the course of normal pregnancy.[20] The pregnant uterus is pear shaped with a narrower lower segment than the fundus and body. The placenta may be implanted anteriorly or posteriorly and wrap

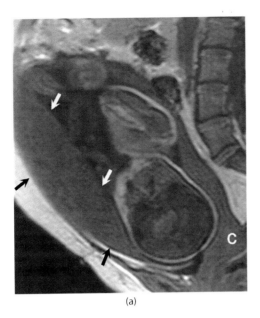
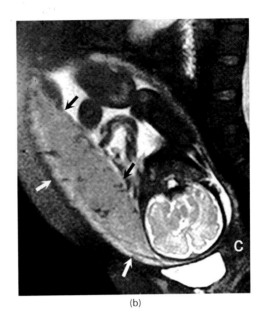

(a)   (b)

FIGURE 4.1   Normal placenta on magnetic resonance imaging (MRI) in the late second trimester. (a) On T1-weighted images, the placenta is homogeneous and isointense to muscle throughout pregnancy. (b) On fat-suppressed T2-weighted images, the placenta is fairly homogeneous and bright with darker thin septa and vessels seen. Note both the inner (fetal) surface (white arrows, a; black arrows, b) and outer (maternal) surface (black arrows, a; white arrows, b) of the placenta are smooth. There is no placenta previa in this case as the anterior placenta is remote from the cervix ("c," a and b). Later in the third trimester, the inner surface may become lobulated in a regular pattern related to the cotyledons; however, the outer maternal surface remains smooth, flowing the expected contour of the uterine wall.

laterally. The lower edge of the placenta is easily visualized, making assessment of the distance between the placental and cervix relatively easy. On T1-weighted images, the placenta appears homogeneous and is isointense to muscle throughout pregnancy. Thus, it is difficult to examine the placental–uterine interface or the myometrium (Figure 4.1a). Fat-suppressed T2-weighted imaging also shows the placenta to be bright and homogeneous in texture with darker thin septae and vessels (Figure 4.1b). The fetal and maternal surfaces of the placenta appear smooth. In the third trimester, the inner fetal surface of the placenta may become lobulated in a pattern related to maturation of the placental cotyledons. The outer maternal surface should remain smooth, following the contours of the uterine wall. When contrast is used, the placenta enhances prior to the myometrium and with increasing age becomes more homogeneous.[21,22] Normal myometrium has a three-layered appearance on T2-weighted images with a heterogeneous hyperintense middle layer and low-intensity margins (Figure 4.1b). As pregnancy progresses, the myometrium thins as the uterus enlarges.

MRI and Placenta Accreta

Over the last 20 years, numerous authors have described MRI features, which suggest possible placenta accreta.[22–28] These include a heterogeneous appearance of the placenta with linear T2-hypointense intra-placental bands, abnormal uterine segment bulging, disruption of the hypo intense bladder wall and a nodular appearance of the bladder outline with placental extension into the bladder. Figure 4.2 shows a placenta with features of accreta. T2-weighted images are shown in sagittal (a) and coronal (b) planes demonstrating a heterogeneous disorganized placental signal with dark T2 bands, an irregular, lobular outer contour, and bladder indentation. Obtaining additional sequences may allow concerning features to be further evaluated. Figure 4.3 shows a case with a posterior placenta previa without accreta. T2-weighted SSFSE images show the interface between the placenta and uterine wall. On T2-weighted images, dark linear structures may represent normal intra-placental vessels or the dark bands associated

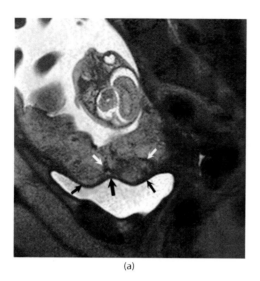
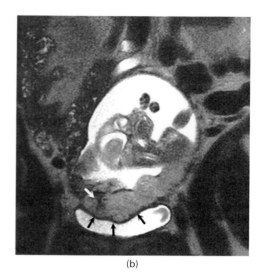

(a)   (b)

FIGURE 4.2 Placenta accreta. Sagittal (a) and coronal (b) T2-weighted images show heterogeneous, disorganized signal, dark T2 bands (white arrows, a and b), and irregular, lobular, outer contour (black arrows, a and b) indenting the partially distended bladder.

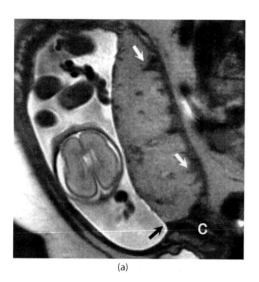
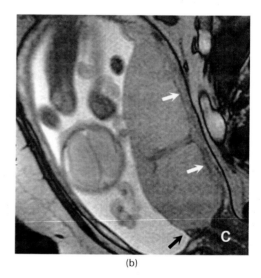

(a)   (b)

FIGURE 4.3 Posterior placenta previa with no accreta: value of FISP/FIESTA sequence. (a) The T2-weighted SSSFE/HASTE shows fairly a homogeneous placenta previa with normal but indistinct interface with the uterine wall. In addition, dark linear structures are seen that may be confused with dark bands of accreta (white arrows, a). (b) On the T2/T1-weighted steady-state gradient echo (FISP/FIESTA), the dark bands are not seen (suggesting they are vascular structures), and it is easier to distinguish placental–maternal interface, which may be seen as a thin dark line (white arrows, b) separating the placenta from the uterine wall. The vascularity of the uterine wall frequently leads to low signal intensity on T2-weighted images and higher signal intensity on FISP/FIESTA images. The anterior placental edge is seen (black arrow, a and b), covering the internal orifice (os) of the cervix ("c," a and b).

with accreta. Often, a T2/T1-weighted steady-state gradient echo sequence helps distinguish between placental bands and vessels; placental bands appear dark on this sequence and vessels appear bright. The placental–uterine interface is often better seen on T2/T1-weighted steady-state gradient echo, appearing as a dark line separating the placenta from the uterine wall. The vascularity of the uterine wall frequently leads to low signal intensity on T2-weighted images and higher signal intensity on FISP/FIESTA images.

MRI and Placenta Accreta and Gestational Age at Evaluation

There is general consensus that MRI to evaluate fetal anatomy is of little use at gestational ages of less than 18 weeks because of the small fetal size and high rate of motion artifact. MRI is of greater use at 20–22 weeks or later depending on the area of interest.[7] An awareness that placenta accreta may be diagnosed with ultrasound as early as the first trimester[29–32] has led to MRI being performed at earlier and earlier gestational ages for confirmation of ultrasound suspected diagnoses. A recent study[33] examined the diagnostic utility of MRI performed at 14–41 weeks gestation. The authors showed that when MRI was performed at less than 24 weeks, the sensitivity and specificity for a diagnosis of placenta accreta was 0.14 and 0.7, respectively. This was considerably worse than the values of 0.79 and 0.94 obtained after 24 weeks. The positive predictive value (PPV) and negative predictive value (NPV) in studies at less than 24 weeks gestation (0.25 and 0.54, respectively) were also worse than after 24 weeks (0.96 and 0.71, respectively). They concluded that MRI evaluation should be delayed until after 24 weeks gestation.

MRI and Provider Experience and Training

MRI evaluation of placental disorders is difficult and requires specialized training and experience. Early reports of MRI diagnosis of placenta accreta were limited to individual cases or small case series often reported by pioneers in the field.[23,24,27,34] A recent meta-analysis of pre-natal diagnosis of invasive placentation included 18 studies containing 1010 pregnancies at risk for placenta accreta.[35] The sensitivity of MRI for diagnosing placenta accreta ranged from 81.3% to 95.1% (mean 90.2%) with a specificity ranging from 76.7% to 94.4% (mean 88.2%). One factor affecting diagnostic performance is observer experience. A recent study[36] showed that more experienced radiologists performed better than junior radiologists in the blind diagnosis of confirmed cases of placenta accreta using the same diagnostic criteria (sensitivity 90.9% specificity 75% for seniors, 81.8% and 61.8% for juniors). They recommended that MRI for the diagnosis of accreta be performed in reference centers with high levels of experience. The use of scoring systems for the diagnostic features of placenta accreta such as that published by Ueno et al.[37] may aid in reducing such inter-observer variation but have not yet been widely tested.

MRI or Ultrasound for Screening and Initial Diagnosis of Placenta Accreta

Several studies examined the performance of MRI versus ultrasound as the primary diagnostic modality for diagnosing placenta accreta.[35,38–41] Ultrasound and MRI performed similarly for primary diagnosis in all studies with no differences found in sensitivity or specificity between the imaging techniques (MRI sensitivity 92.9%, US sensitivity 87.8%, $p = 0.24$; MRI specificity 93.5%, US specificity 96.3%, $p = 0.91$).[35]

Given the relative availability, ease of performance, and lower cost of ultrasound versus MRI, it follows that ultrasound should be the primary screening tool for accreta in at-risk patients. The details of ultrasound evaluation of placenta accreta are reviewed in detail in Chapter 3.

MRI and Antepartum Hemorrhage

Bleeding in pregnancy should be evaluated initially with ultrasound. This is particularly true in the second half of pregnancy where placenta previa should always be excluded prior to vaginal examination. In cases where accreta is suspected in the setting of bleeding in a hemodynamically stable patient, MRI may have a diagnostic role. Figure 4.4a shows a sagittal T2-weighted image of a placenta accreta with outer bulging of the placenta, and Figure 4.4b shows a T2/T1-weighted FISP/FIESTA image. Both figures suggest that there is placental tissue at the internal orifice (os). The T1-weighted image in Figure 4.4c clearly shows that this apparent placental tissue is an area of hemorrhage, demonstrating the value of such additional sequences.

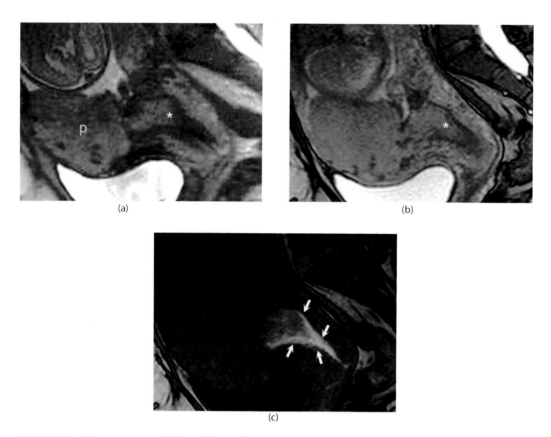

FIGURE 4.4 Placenta accreta with hemorrhage: value of T1-weighted sequence. (a) Sagittal T2-weighted image shows placenta accreta ("p," a) with outer bulging of the placenta. Note the material at the internal os has the appearance of placental tissue on both T2-weighted (a) and T2/T1-weighted FISP/FIESTA (b) images ("*," a and b). On the T1-weighted image (c), we see there is hemorrhage in this location (arrows, c). This case demonstrates the importance of a T1-weighted sequence to clearly identify blood products that may mimic solid tissue on other sequences.

MRI for Assessment of Depth of Myometrial Invasion

The gold standard for assessment of the depth of placental invasion is histopathology. It should be noted, however, that in a single specimen, varying degrees of placental invasion from accreta, increta, and percreta may occur, depending on the site examined. Ultrasound has been shown to have a wide range of diagnostic confidence in determining degree of placental invasion from 38% to 65%.[42,43] Figure 4.5a shows a sagittal T2-weighted image of placenta accreta with outer bulging of the placenta and invasion into the cervix. Figure 4.5b shows the axial T2-weighted view (oriented axial to the cervix) with the dark inner fibrous stromal ring of the cervix replaced by the invasive placenta anteriorly. Figures 4.5c and 4.5d show a normal intact appearance of the dark fibrous stroma in a normal cervix. The previously cited meta-analysis of MRI and placenta accreta[35] found a sensitivity of 92.9% (72.8%–99.5%) and a specificity of 97.6% (87.1%–99.9%) for depth of myometrial invasion. Palacios-Jaraquemada described a system of classifying degree of placental invasion coupled with topographic assessment of the placenta in 300 cases[44] and reported accurate assessment of placental invasion in 97.66% of cases with a 1.33% false positive rate and 1% false negative rate. This system was applied retrospectively to 62 patients managed at a single center.[43] Partial myometrial invasion was graded A, invasion to full thickness of myometrium B, and invasion into parametrium or cervix C. The location of invasion was classified as S1, upper uterine segment supplied by uterine and upper vesical arteries, and S2, lower uterine segment supplied by deep anastomotic pelvic subperitoneal vessels. Severity ranged from S1A

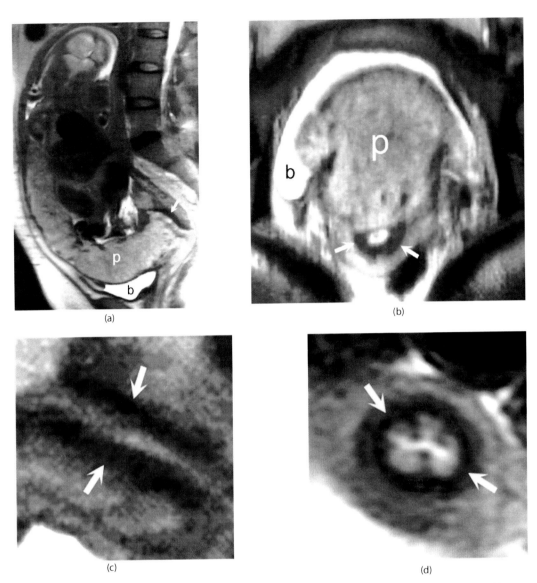

FIGURE 4.5 Placenta accreta with cervical invasion. (a) Sagittal T2-weighted image shows placenta accreta with outer bulging of the placenta ("p," a) and invasion into the cervix; only the posterior dark stripe of normal fibrous stroma is seen (arrow, a). (b) On the axial T2-weighted view, the dark inner fibrous stromal ring (arrows, b) of the cervix is partially replaced by the anterior invasive placenta ("p," b). Note relationship of the placenta with fluid in the bladder ("b," a and b). (c) For comparison, sagittal (c) and axial (d) T2-weighted images indicate the normal intact appearance of the dark fibrous stroma of the cervix (arrows, c and d).

(least severe) to S2C (most severe). MRI assessment was compared to pathological and surgical staging. The authors reported a 61% rate of accuracy for staging, with a 22.6% rate of over diagnosis of degree of invasion. Further prospective studies are needed to examine the true utility of this approach.

MRI as a Tie Breaker in Uncertain Diagnosis of Accreta

In cases where it is difficult to determine if an accreta is present, MRI may be useful as an adjunctive diagnostic test. This may be particularly true in cases of posterior placentation, especially in later gestation when it is difficult to visualize the placenta by sonogram, or suspected accreta absent of placenta previa. Such difficult cases may also benefit from the use of contrast media.

MRI with Gadolinium Contrast

The dark T2 bands seen with placenta accreta were initially thought to represent fibrous tissue. Figure 4.6a shows these dark bands on a sagittal T2-weighted image. Figure 4.6b is a delayed gadolinium-enhanced T1-weighted image showing that the bands do not enhance even after some delay as would be expected of fibrous tissue. These dark bands probably represent infarcts and are indicative of accreta.

Figure 4.7 compares a placenta previa without accreta (a,b) and a placenta previa with accreta (c,d). Figures 4.7a,c are T2-weighted images while Figures 4.7a,d are delayed gadolinium-enhanced T1-weighted images. The non-invasive placenta (Figure 4.7a) shows a smooth outer uterine contour and outlining of the placental–internal interface, and the contrast enhanced image (Figure 4.7b) shows maternal vessels seen beneath the placental tissue. The placenta accreta (Figures 4.7b,d) shows bulging of the outer uterine margin, a heterogeneous placenta with multiple non-enhancing dark T2 bands and no maternal vessels between the placenta and bladder fluid. Signal intensity on T2-weighted images and contrast enhancement appears more heterogeneous and disorganized in invasive compared to normal placenta.

Incorporation of MRI into a Diagnostic and Management Paradigm for Placenta Accreta

Patients at increased risk of placenta accreta should initially be screened using ultrasound.[12] Those with suspicious findings should be referred for confirmatory evaluation by an experienced observer. Inconclusive ultrasound findings should be followed by MRI evaluation.[45] Cases where diagnosis remains equivocal after ultrasound and non-contrast MRI may merit evaluation with contrast-enhanced MRI.[9] MRI may add little to the initial diagnosis of placenta accreta but may have a role in staging and

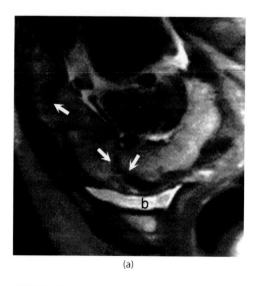
(a)

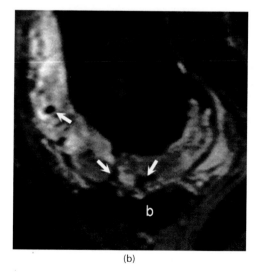
(b)

FIGURE 4.6 Placenta accreta: dark T2 bands. It was initially thought that the dark T2 bands may represent fibrous tissue; however, in this example dark bands on sagittal T2-weighted (a) and delayed gadolinium-enhanced T1-weighted (b) images show that they do not enhance even after some delay (arrows, a and b). Delayed enhancement would be expected of fibrous tissue. These likely represent infarcts. Note indentation of the placenta upon the bladder ("b," a and b).

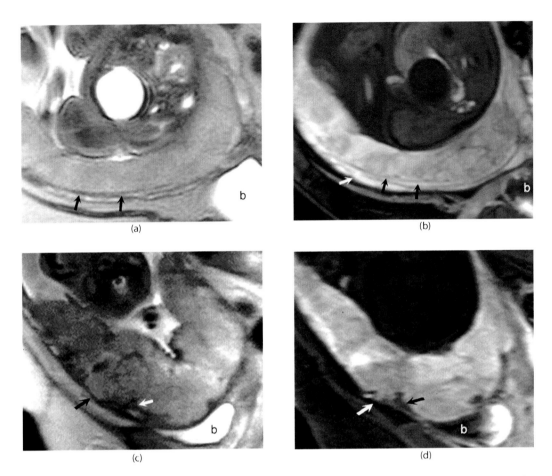

FIGURE 4.7 Placental enhancement: normal versus placenta accreta. Sagittal T2-weighted (a and c) and delayed gado-linium enhanced T1-weighted images (b and d) in a normal placenta (a and b) and placenta accreta (c and d). Both patients have anterior placenta previa. In the non-invasive placenta (a and b), the outer uterine contour is smooth (black arrows, a and b), the placenta–maternal interface is outlined and on enhanced images maternal vessels are seen beneath the placental tissue (white arrow, b). In the invasive placenta (c and d), the outer uterine margin shows bulging (black arrow, c; white arrow, d), the placenta is heterogeneous, with multiple non-enhancing dark T2 bands (white arrow, c; black arrow, d) and no maternal vessels are seen between the placental tissue and fluid within the bladder ("b," a through d).

determining options for surgical management.[43,44] MRI assessment of the degree of placental invasion into the myometrium and extension into the parametrium appears to be superior to ultrasound assessment and may aid in determining the likely complexity and morbidity of surgery or the feasibility of uterine conservation. In turn, this may inform decisions as to whether to plan a cesarean hysterectomy or attempt placental removal, as well as to plan for appropriate surgical expertise if bladder and ureteral surgery is required.

REFERENCES

1. Johnson IR, Symonds EM, Kean DM et al. Imaging the pregnant human uterus with nuclear magnetic resonance. *Am J Obstet Gynecol.* 1984;148(8):1136–1139.
2. Smith FW, MacLennan F, Abramovich DR, MacGilivray I, Hutchison JM. NMR imaging in human pregnancy: A preliminary study. *Magn Reson Imaging.* 1984;2(1):57–64.
3. McCarthy SM, Filly RA, Stark DD et al. Obstetrical magnetic resonance imaging: Fetal anatomy. *Radiology.* 1985;154(2):427–432.

4. Powell MC, Buckley J, Price H, Worthington BS, Symonds EM. Magnetic resonance imaging and placenta previa. *Am J Obstet Gynecol.* 1986;154(3):565–569.

5. Levine D. Obstetric MRI. *J Magn Reson Imaging.* 2006;24(1):1–15.

6. Levine D, Barnes PD, Edelman RR. Obstetric MR imaging. *Radiology.* 1999;211(3):609–617.

7. Reddy UM, Abuhamad AZ, Levine D, Saade GR, Fetal Imaging Workshop Invited Participants. Fetal imaging: Executive summary of a joint Eunice Kennedy Shriver National Institute of Child Health and Human Development, Society for Maternal-Fetal Medicine, American Institute of Ultrasound in Medicine, American College of Obstetricians and Gynecologists, American College of Radiology, Society for Pediatric Radiology, and Society of Radiologists in Ultrasound Fetal Imaging Workshop. *Obstet Gynecol.* 2014;123(5):1070–1082.

8. Expert Panel on MRS, Kanal E, Barkovich AJ. ACR guidance document on MR safe practices: 2013. *J Magn Reson Imaging.* 2013;37(3):501–530.

9. American College of Obstetricians and Gynecologists' Committee on Obstetric Practice. Committee opinion No. 656: Guidelines for diagnostic imaging during pregnancy and lactation. *Obstet Gynecol.* 2016;127(2):e75–e80.

10. Chen MM, Coakley FV, Kaimal A, Laros RK Jr. Guidelines for computed tomography and magnetic resonance imaging use during pregnancy and lactation. *Obstet Gynecol.* 2008;112(2 Pt 1):333–340.

11. Wataganara T, Ebrashy A, Aliyu LD et al. Fetal magnetic resonance imaging and ultrasound. *J Perinat Med.* 2016;44:533–542.

12 Committee on Obstetric Practice. Committee opinion no. 529: Placenta accreta. *Obstet Gynecol.* 2012;120(1):207–211.

13. Webb JA, Thomsen HS, Morcos SK, Members of Contrast Media Safety Committee of European Society of Urogenital Radiology. The use of iodinated and gadolinium contrast media during pregnancy and lactation. *Eur Radiol.* 2005;15(6):1234–1240.

14. De Santis M, Straface G, Cavaliere AF, Carducci B, Caruso A. Gadolinium periconceptional exposure: Pregnancy and neonatal outcome. *Acta Obstet Gynecol Scand.* 2007;86(1):99–101.

15. Webb JA, Thomsen HS. Gadolinium contrast media during pregnancy and lactation. *Acta Radiol.* 2013;54(6):599–600.

16. Thomsen HS, Morcos SK, Almen T et al. Nephrogenic systemic fibrosis and gadolinium-based contrast media: Updated ESUR Contrast Medium Safety Committee guidelines. *Eur Radiol.* 2013;23(2):307–318.

17. Oh KY, Roberts VH, Schabel MC, Grove KL, Woods M, Frias AE. Gadolinium chelate contrast material in pregnancy: Fetal biodistribution in the nonhuman primate. *Radiology.* 2015;276(1):110–118.

18. Allen BC, Leyendecker JR. Placental evaluation with magnetic resonance. *Radiol Clin North Am.* 2013;51(6):955–966.

19. Masselli G, Gualdi G. MR imaging of the placenta: What a radiologist should know. *Abdom Imaging.* 2013;38(3):573–587.

20. Blaicher W, Brugger PC, Mittermayer C et al. Magnetic resonance imaging of the normal placenta. *Eur J Radiol.* 2006;57(2):256–260.

21. Marcos HB, Semelka RC, Worawattanakul S. Normal placenta: Gadolinium-enhanced dynamic MR imaging. *Radiology.* 1997;205(2):493–496.

22. Tanaka YO, Sohda S, Shigemitsu S, Niitsu M, Itai Y. High temporal resolution dynamic contrast MRI in a high risk group for placenta accreta. *Magn Reson Imaging.* 2001;19(5):635–642.

23. Thorp JM Jr., Councell RB, Sandridge DA, Wiest HH. Antepartum diagnosis of placenta previa percreta by magnetic resonance imaging. *Obstet Gynecol.* 1992;80(3 Pt 2):506–508.

24. Fejgin MD, Rosen DJ, Ben-Nun I, Goldberger SB, Beyth Y. Ultrasonic and magnetic resonance imaging diagnosis of placenta accreta managed conservatively. *J Perinat Med.* 1993;21(2):165–168.

25. Levine D, Hulka CA, Ludmir J, Li W, Edelman RR. Placenta accreta: Evaluation with color Doppler US, power Doppler US, and MR imaging. *Radiology.* 1997;205(3):773–776.

26. Ha TP, Li KC. Placenta accreta: MRI antenatal diagnosis and surgical correlation. *J Magn Reson Imaging.* 1998;8(3):748–750.

27. Maldjian C, Adam R, Pelosi M, Pelosi M, 3rd, Rudelli RD, Maldjian J. MRI appearance of placenta percreta and placenta accreta. *Magn Reson Imaging.* 1999;17(7):965–971.

28. Lax A, Prince MR, Mennitt KW, Schwebach JR, Budorick NE. The value of specific MRI features in the evaluation of suspected placental invasion. *Magn Reson Imaging.* 2007;25(1):87–93.

29. Chen YJ, Wang PH, Liu WM, Lai CR, Shu LP, Hung JH. Placenta accreta diagnosed at 9 weeks' gestation. *Ultrasound Obstet Gynecol.* 2002;19(6):620–622.

30. Wong HS, Zuccollo J, Tait J, Pringle KC. Placenta accreta in the first trimester of pregnancy: Sonographic findings. *J Clin Ultrasound.* 2009;37(2):100–103.

31. Ballas J, Pretorius D, Hull AD, Resnik R, Ramos GA. Identifying sonographic markers for placenta accreta in the first trimester. *J Ultrasound Med.* 2012;31(11):1835–1841.

32. Stirnemann JJ, Mousty E, Chalouhi G, Salomon LJ, Bernard JP, Ville Y. Screening for placenta accreta at 11–14 weeks of gestation. *Am J Obstet Gynecol.* 2011;205(6):547.e1–e6.

33. Horowitz JM, Berggruen S, McCarthy RJ et al. When timing is everything: Are placental MRI examinations performed before 24 weeks' gestational age reliable? *Am J Roentgenol.* 2015;205(3):685–692.

34. Comstock CH. Antenatal diagnosis of placenta accreta: A review. *Ultrasound Obstet Gynecol.* 2005;26(1):89–96.

35. D'Antonio F, Iacovella C, Palacios-Jaraquemada J, Bruno CH, Manzoli L, Bhide A. Prenatal identification of invasive placentation using magnetic resonance imaging: Systematic review and meta-analysis. *Ultrasound Obstet Gynecol.* 2014;44(1):8–16.

36. Alamo L, Anaye A, Rey J. Detection of suspected placental invasion by MRI: Do the results depend on observers' experience? *Eur J Radiol.* 2013;82(2):e51–e57.

37. Ueno Y, Maeda T, Tanaka U et al. Evaluation of interobserver variability and diagnostic performance of developed MRI-based radiological scoring system for invasive placenta previa. *J Magn Reson Imaging.* 2016;44:573–583.

38. Riteau AS, Tassin M, Chambon G et al. Accuracy of ultrasonography and magnetic resonance imaging in the diagnosis of placenta accreta. *PLoS One.* 2014;9(4):e94866.

39. Algebally AM, Yousef RR, Badr SS, Al Obeidly A, Szmigielski W, Al Ibrahim AA. The value of ultrasound and magnetic resonance imaging in diagnostics and prediction of morbidity in cases of placenta previa with abnormal placentation. *Pol J Radiol.* 2014;79:409–416.

40. Rezk MA, Shawky M. Grey-scale and colour Doppler ultrasound versus magnetic resonance imaging for the prenatal diagnosis of placenta accreta. *J Matern Fetal Neonatal Med.* 2016;29(2):218–223.

41. Satija B, Kumar S, Wadhwa L et al. Utility of ultrasound and magnetic resonance imaging in prenatal diagnosis of placenta accreta: A prospective study. *Indian J Radiol Imaging.* 2015;25(4):464–470.

42. Bowman ZS, Eller AG, Kennedy AM et al. Accuracy of ultrasound for the prediction of placenta accreta. *Am J Obstet Gynecol.* 2014;211(2):177.e1–e7.

43. Aitken K, Allen L, Pantazi S et al. MRI Significantly improves disease staging to direct surgical planning for abnormal invasive placentation: A single centre experience. *J Obstet Gynaecol Can.* 2016;38(3):246–251.e1.

44. Palacios Jaraquemada JM, Bruno CH. Magnetic resonance imaging in 300 cases of placenta accreta: Surgical correlation of new findings. *Acta Obstet Gynecol Scand.* 2005;84(8):716–724.

45. Warshak CR, Eskander R, Hull AD et al. Accuracy of ultrasonography and magnetic resonance imaging in the diagnosis of placenta accreta. *Obstet Gynecol.* 2006;108(3 Pt 1):573–581.

5

Optimal Timing of Delivery of Placenta Accreta

Carolyn Haunschild and Deirdre Lyell

CONTENTS

Introduction

In contrast to days when placenta accreta, increta, and percreta (from here referred to as placenta accreta, unless otherwise noted) were diagnosed only at delivery, prenatal diagnosis of suspected accreta has created the need for the physician to decide when and where to deliver. Despite the increased incidence of placenta accreta during the past several decades, now occurring in as many as 1 in 533 to 1 in 272 deliveries,[1,2] it remains uncommon enough that high-quality data are lacking for many aspects of management, and there is discordance between delivery timing recommendations[3] and delivery timing in practice.[4,5] This chapter discusses guidance recommendations for delivery timing, the basis and limitations of such recommendations, and what is done in practice.

National Institute of Child Health and Human Development (NICHD) and Society for Maternal–Fetal Medicine (SMFM) Delivery Timing Guidance

The Eunice Kennedy Shriver NICHD and SMFM convened a workshop in 2011 to address timing of indicated late preterm birth, from which experts developed delivery timing guidelines for many conditions including suspected placenta accreta with placenta previa.[3] Experts developed a consensus opinion based on available data and opinion, weighing the maternal, fetal, and neonatal risks and benefits of

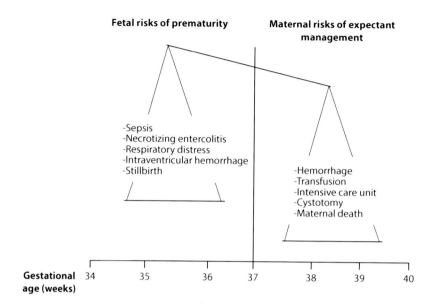

FIGURE 5.1 As gestational age increases, the maternal risks of expectant management of placenta accreta begin to outweigh the fetal risks of prematurity. (Adapted from Spong CY et al. *Obstet Gynecol*, 118, 323–233, 2011.)

ongoing pregnancy versus delivery. Based on what they judged to be limited or inconsistent scientific evidence, the experts issued a guideline that women with suspected placenta accreta *with* placenta previa be delivered between 34 0/7 and 35 6/7 weeks (Figure 5.1).[3]

The authors acknowledged several key factors in issuing this guideline.[3] With suspected placenta accreta with previa, the goals of late-preterm delivery are to avoid catastrophic maternal complications (primarily from maternal hemorrhage and its sequelae), to limit the potential for fetal death or compromise from prematurity or maternal hemorrhage, and to avoid an unscheduled delivery performed in a non-ideal location or under suboptimal circumstances. An unscheduled delivery for maternal hemorrhage can result in maternal morbidity and fetal or neonatal hypoxemia or acidemia resulting from maternal hypovolemic shock; delivery in a nonideal location can result in decreased availability of needed critical resources such as blood products, dedicated operating room staff, and surgical specialists.

The guideline was not intended to serve as a standard of care. The authors acknowledged the importance of individualized clinical management that incorporates individual maternal and fetal risks, comorbidities, available resources of the practice setting, and patient preferences. Factors guiding delivery timing recommendations, particularly risk estimates of the major maternal and neonatal morbidities, and limitations of the data, are discussed in the following sections.

Factors Guiding Delivery Timing Recommendations

The risk of massive hemorrhage at delivery or during pregnancy among women with previa and accreta is thought to increase with gestational age.[3,6–8] Delivery timing recommendations must weigh the morbidities and risks of hemorrhage, and the risk of emergent delivery due to hemorrhage versus scheduled delivery, including the risks of delivery in a suboptimal location.

Limitations of Data

Most studies are relatively small, retrospective, utilize a cohort with postdelivery confirmation of accreta rather than predelivery suspicion (when delivery decisions need to be made), often combine outcomes for women with previa with accreta and previa without accreta, and do not control for the many nuances that often determine patient outcome. These include severity of the suspected accreta, quality of antenatal detection, availability of in-house physicians, and delivery circumstance. Further, much is unknown about accreta itself, including whether the degree of invasion progresses with time, and predelivery prediction of severity is limited. Finally, predictors of hemorrhage in placenta accreta with previa are often extrapolated from studies of women with previa alone.

There are currently no randomized controlled trials (RCTs) or well-controlled observational studies to guide best practices in delivery timing.[9] Until such an RCT is conducted, recommendations for prospective decisions about delivery timing must be extrapolated from imperfect data, with an attempt to balance difficult to predict and potentially catastrophic maternal risks of expectant management with its intended benefit, improved neonatal outcome.

Maternal Hemorrhage, Delivery Timing, Prediction, and Risk

Postpartum hemorrhage is the most frequent root cause of maternal morbidity and mortality in placenta accreta and are discussed here.[10]

Maternal Hemorrhage and Its Sequelae

As discussed elsewhere in this book, abnormal placentation confers a higher odds of a severe postpartum hemorrhage than any other etiology, even when adjusting for confounders.[10] Average blood loss at delivery among women with placenta accreta with previa is estimated at 2,000–3,000 mL.[5,11,12] Ninety to ninety-five percent of women undergoing hysterectomy for placenta accreta receive a blood transfusion.[6,13] Five to forty percent of cases require massive transfusion of 10 units of red blood cells or more,[6,7,13] with similar transfusion requirements noted among women with accreta, increta, and percreta.[6,13] Hemorrhage can lead to hypoxic encephalopathy, acute tubular necrosis, and acute respiratory distress syndrome (RDS). Both hemorrhage and transfusion can lead to coagulopathy and disseminated intravascular coagulation. Transfusion is also associated with transfusion-related acute lung injury. Such massive transfusion at delivery, as well as the potential surgical complexity of the delivery, has led many to advocate for early, scheduled delivery. [6,8,14–16]

Timing of Hemorrhage

The risk of bleeding from placenta previa alone is thought to increase with advancing gestation,[3,8,17] with risk of emergent bleeding precipitating delivery estimated at 4.7% at 35 weeks, 15% by 36 weeks, 30% by 37 weeks, and 59% by 38 weeks.[17,18] Based on reported increasing risks of bleeding, the NICHD/SMFM guideline recommends delivering women with uncomplicated placenta previa between 36 0/7 and 37 6/7 weeks.[3]

Most authors report an increased risk of bleeding with advancing gestation among women with placenta accreta or percreta.[3,6–8,14,19] Warshak et al. reported that outcomes among 62 women with predelivery suspicion for placenta accreta and postoperative pathologic confirmation, in a setting where "cesarean hysterectomy typically was scheduled between 34 and 35 weeks."[14] Among the 62 women, 22 (35%) required emergent delivery before their scheduled date, most frequently for bleeding (18 [22%]), as well as contractions (1 [5%]) and nonreassuring fetal heart rate (3 [14%]). Among nine women who were not scheduled earlier and did not require delivery prior to 36 weeks, four (44%) required emergent delivery for hemorrhage. Bowman et al.[19] reported a 31% rate of delivery for bleeding prior to a scheduled 36-week delivery among 77 women, with 12% delivering early due to labor.

Similarly, Al-Kahn et al. reported retrospective outcomes of 67 women with placenta accreta identified through computerized records from the pathology department from a 10-year period. During the second 5 years of the study period, deliveries were planned at 34 weeks (42 women total). Among women with a targeted delivery date of 34 weeks, delivery occurred prior to 34 weeks due to bleeding among 21%, and due to preterm premature rupture of membranes (PPROM) among 8%.[7] In a letter to the editor, Meller et al.[20] reported outcomes among 95 women with suspected placenta accreta managed during a 10-year period, of whom 83% ($n = 79$) had postnatal confirmation of placenta accreta. The group achieved a scheduled delivery goal of 36 weeks among 67% (*n* = 53) of the cohort. The remaining 33% (*n* = 26) delivered at a mean gestational age of 30.9 ± 4.5 weeks, primarily due to vaginal bleeding (*n* = 23).

The highest rate of delivery due to hemorrhage is reported from a survey on placenta percreta that was conducted among of members of the Society for Perinatal Obstetricians in 1995.[6] After 35 weeks' gestation, bleeding was the indication for delivery in 93% of reported cases. Four of eight maternal deaths occurred after 36 weeks.

Robinson and Grobman[8] created a decision analysis to determine the optimal gestational age for delivery in women with placenta previa with sonographic evidence of placenta accreta. The authors estimated the risks for maternal hemorrhage, perinatal mortality, and intensive care unit (ICU) admission, weighted outcomes including maternal ICU admission, neonatal RDS, cerebral palsy, mental retardation, and infant death, and then modeled outcomes for nine strategies for delivery between 34 and 39 weeks (with and without steroids at 34 and 35 weeks, and with and without lung maturity amniocentesis at 36–38 weeks). The strategy with the highest quality-adjusted life years and the preferred strategy in most situations was planned delivery at 34 weeks after administration of antenatal corticosteroids, without confirmation of fetal lung maturity. However, when the risk of antepartum hemorrhage at 34 weeks is between 1% and 7%, the preferred strategy is delivery at 37 weeks' gestation. Unfortunately, the quantification of individual risk for catastrophic antepartum hemorrhage is limited (Table 5.1).

In contrast to studies that identify a 21%–93% rate of emergent delivery due to hemorrhage by 34–35 weeks in women with suspected accreta, a recent retrospective cohort study reported lower rates of antepartum hemorrhage by gestational age among women with placenta accreta and with previa alone.[5] Standard practice in the authors' institution is to deliver women with suspected accreta at 36–38 weeks.[5] By week, urgent delivery for bleeding among women with sonographic suspicion for placenta accreta occurred among 2.5% before 34 weeks, 10% between 34 and 35 6/7 weeks, 7.6% between 36 and 37 6/7 weeks, and 1.3% at 38 weeks or greater, with cumulative totals of 12.5% by 36 weeks, 20.1% by 38 weeks, and 24.4% at 38 weeks and beyond. Among women with postdelivery confirmation of placenta accreta, as opposed to sonographic suspicion, 6%, 11%, 29%, 54%, and 71% were delivered for any reason by 34, 35, 36, 37, and 38 weeks of gestation, respectively.[5] The authors concluded that approximately 90% of women with placenta accreta can be delivered after 36 weeks' gestation without a bleeding complication.[5] It is important to note that all of these studies were conducted in large tertiary care centers with extensive 24/7 in-house support.

Predictors of Maternal Hemorrhage

Accurate prediction of which women are at risk for the greatest degrees of hemorrhage could help determine who should undergo early delivery earlier versus expectant management. However, prospective

TABLE 5.1

Decision Analysis of Various Delivery Strategies for Placenta Previa Accreta. The Recommended Delivery Strategy is a 34-Weeks Gestational Age after Steroid Administration

Weeks GA	RR of Maternal Hemorrhage Requiring Delivery	RR of RDS	RR of Infant Mortality	QALY	Rank
34[a]	0.18*	0.064*	0.00379*	119.31	1
35[a]	1.0	0.50	0.864	119.17	2
36[b]	1.4	0.50	0.673	119.05	3
37[b]	1.96	0.07	0.383	118.99	4
38[b]	1.96	0.0055	0.372	118.86	5
39[b]	–	0.003	0.216	118.74	6

Abbreviations: GA, gestational age; RR, relative risk; RDS, respiratory distress syndrome; QALY, quality-adjusted life year.
*Referent value
[a]After steroid administration.
[b]The QALY with amniocentesis for fetal lung maturity testing consistently ranks lower than without amniocentesis and is generally not recommended. It has been omitted as a strategy from this table.

predictors of hemorrhage are limited and the unheralded nature of potentially catastrophic maternal hemorrhage is the rationale for early scheduled delivery.

Cervical Length

Several groups found that shorter cervical length (CL) in placenta previa is associated with more bleeding episodes during pregnancy and with earlier delivery due to hemorrhage.[21-25] While no CL cut-off is absolutely predictive of delivery or safe expectant management, these studies may help identify which women with placenta previa, and by extrapolation placenta previa with accreta, are at greater risk for emergent delivery.

CL of ≤30 mm at 32 weeks has been associated with an increased risk of hemorrhage and emergent delivery.[21] In 68 women with placenta previa at 32 weeks, a transvaginal CL of 30 mm or less was associated with delivery for hemorrhage (79% vs. 28%, $p < 0.001$) and emergent delivery (76% vs. 28%, $p < 0.001$). Women with a short cervix (≤30 mm) were more likely to undergo hospitalization for bleeding during pregnancy and to experience symptomatic contractions; their risk for preterm delivery was increased by more than threefold. Vaginal bleeding itself was associated with both a short cervix and contractions. When the CL was >30 mm, 64% of women did not experience bleeding episodes, hospitalization, and delivered at term. The incidence of a short cervix among the entire cohort was high (29 women [43%]). In a logistic regression analysis, the probability of hemorrhage requiring delivery ranged from as low as 10%–20% for CLs of 50–60 mm to as high as 60%–100% for CLs <10–15 mm.[21] Given that 28% of women with a CL >30 mm still required emergent delivery for hemorrhage, the greatest utility of CL for prediction hemorrhage may lie at the extremes when determining timing of delivery for women with placenta accreta (Table 5.2).

Similarly, others also found a correlation between short cervix and hemorrhage prompting preterm cesarean delivery. One plausible hypothesis is that parturition, broadening of the lower uterine segment, and dilation of the internal orifice (os) during the third trimester causes hemorrhage, and likely correlates with cervical shortening.[25] In a retrospective study of 71 women with placenta previa who underwent serial CL evaluation every 2 weeks, Sekiguchi et al. found that the odds ratio (OR) for preterm cesarean delivery for hemorrhage based on CL ≤35 was 4.67.[23] Zaitoun et al. found that more women with CL <30 mm underwent emergency cesarean delivery <34 weeks (16[89%] vs. 4[21%] with CL ≥30 mm, $p = 0.004$).[24] Fukushima et al. categorized women with placenta previa based on CL >30 mm or ≤30 mm. Women with CL ≤30 mm were more likely to undergo emergent cesarean delivery prior to 37 weeks.[25]

In contrast, in one small study of CL among women undergoing cesarean hysterectomy for placenta percreta with previa, CL did not correlate with gestational age at delivery.[26] When a breakpoint of CL ≤20.5 or >20.5 was assessed, the mean gestational age at delivery among was similar between groups (35.7 weeks [±2.6] for CL ≤20.5 mm, $n = 32$ vs. 34.7 weeks [±2.9] CL >20.5 mm, $n = 29$ women). Surgeries were routinely scheduled between 34 0/7 weeks and 36 6/7 weeks, and delivery decisions were based on patient and placental factors. Of note, CL ≤20.5 mm correlated with transfusion of ≥4 units of erythrocyte/fresh-frozen plasma units perhaps, as the authors speculate, due to a wider lower uterine segment at surgery that caused more hemorrhage.[26]

TABLE 5.2

Outcomes of Placenta Previa Based on a Cervical Length (CL) Cutoff of 30 mm

Study	Cervical Length	Gestational Age (weeks) at Delivery[a]	Emergent Cesarean Section (%)[b]	Maternal Hemorrhage (%)	Mean Birthweight (g)
Stafford et al.[21]	>30 mm vs. <30 mm	>37 vs. 3–36*	28 vs. 76*	28 vs. 79*	2,921 vs. 2,524*
Zaitoun et al.[24]	>30 mm vs. <30 mm	35.6 vs. 33.0*	11 vs. 46*	–	2,800 vs. 1,900*
Fukushima et al.[25]	>30 mm vs. <30 mm	37.1 vs. 36.7*	23 vs. 50*	18 vs. 60*	2,662 vs. 2,560

*$p < 0.05$

[a] Median for Stafford, Mean for Zaitoun and Fukushima.

[b] Unspecified Stafford, before 36 weeks Zaitoun, before 37 weeks Fukushoma.

Antenatal Diagnosis

Data are conflicting on whether antenatal diagnosis of accreta predicts maternal hemorrhage.[11,12,16,27-29] This discrepancy may be due to lack of accounting for differences in accreta subtype, inherent differences in patients, clinical management, and sonographic accuracy.

In a study of 134 cases of placenta accreta in Britain, antenatal diagnosis conferred no difference in the median estimated blood loss (EBL) or transfusion volume, although there was a trend toward more blood loss >2,500 mL among women without antenatal diagnosis.[30] In subgroup analysis of women with suspected placenta increta and percreta, antenatal diagnosis was associated with significantly less blood loss (2,750 mL) compared to unsuspected cases (6,100 mL),[30] likely in part due to a change in surgeon behavior based on expectation of the diagnosis. Women with antenatal suspicion for any of the accreta subtypes were more likely to undergo therapies to prevent hemorrhage (artery embolization, balloon tamponade) whereas those not suspected antenatally were more likely to undergo therapies to treat hemorrhage (uterotonics, intrauterine balloons).[30] Others have shown that women with more clinically significant accretas are more likely to be identified by antenatal diagnosis.[11] Similarly, in a Scandinavian study, among 44 women with placenta accreta, those with an antenatal diagnosis experienced significantly less blood loss (4,500 mL) than those diagnosed intrapartum (7,500 mL).[27]

Others have shown increased blood loss with antenatal diagnosis of accreta. In a retrospective review of pathologically confirmed accreta,[16] women with suspicion for placenta accreta had a greater rate of massive hemorrhage (EBL >5,000) than did women who were not diagnosed on antenatal ultrasound (42% vs. 12%). A retrospective study by the NICHD Maternal–Fetal Medicine Units Network showed that women with morbidly adherent placenta suspected before delivery were more likely to have more EBL >2,750, higher rates of transfusion, and more frequent hysterectomy than unsuspected cases (Table 5.3).[11]

Some have speculated that women with more invasive placenta accretas, as opposed to focal accretas, are more likely to be detected prenatally and also are more likely to experience massive hemorrhage,[12] potentially explaining variability in study outcomes. Al-Khan et al. showed that antenatal diagnosis allowed for predelivery planning in only 31% of pathology-confirmed placenta accretas, but 69% of placenta incretas and 85% of placenta percretas.[7]

However, data are also conflicting regarding the degree of hemorrhage based on accreta subtype. Some studies have shown that women with placenta percreta are more likely to require additional blood products,[29] while several others show no difference in massive hemorrhage for placenta accreta versus increta/percreta.[12,13,21]

Antenatal suspicion for accreta is necessary to allow for decision-making regarding timing of delivery in suspected accreta. However, many outcome studies include accretas only diagnosed after delivery, potentially skewing outcomes toward what may appear to be a lower risk if antenatal diagnosis is

TABLE 5.3

Placenta Accreta Detected Antenatally Is Associated with Higher Estimated Blood Loss and Hysterectomy

Maternal Outcome	Antenatal Suspicion (N = 84)	No antenatal suspicion (N = 74)	*p*-Value
Patients requiring ICU admission	33 (39.3%)	16 (21.6%)	0.02
Total EBL	2,000 mL (1,300–3,000)	1,500 mL (1,000–2,500)	0.004
EBL < 1,100	12 (15%)	24 (32.4%)	–
EBL 1,100–1,899	19 (23.8)	21 (28.4)	–
EBL 1,900–2,749	23 (28.8%)	15 (20.3%)	–
EBL > 2,749	26 (32.5%)	14 (18.9%)	–
Patients requiring transfusion of blood products	67 (79.8%)	38 (51.4%)	<0.001
Patients requiring hysterectomy	77 (91.7%)	33 (44.6%)	<0.001

Abbreviations: EBL, estimated blood loss; ICU, intensive care unit.

indeed associated with more severe cases. Alternatively, the more obvious accreta subtypes diagnosed antenatally may be subject to more aggressive measures, reducing overall blood loss, yet may be prone to greater blood loss overall. In contrast, less severe cases without prenatal diagnosis lose more blood as uterine salvage is attempted, increasing overall blood loss prior to cesarean hysterectomy. This issue demonstrates the heterogeneity of cases and potential outcomes, and the complexity and limitations that also may factor into data on which delivery timing decisions are based. These issues underscore the need for standard and uniform definitions among studies. They also leave the question of whether antenatal diagnosis is associated with more or less maternal hemorrhage unanswered.

Predictors of Unscheduled Delivery

In an institution where delivery in the setting of suspected placenta accreta is scheduled at approximately 36 weeks, Bowman et al.[19] found that among women without vaginal bleeding, contractions, or PPROM, 26/26 women reached 36 weeks' gestation without emergent delivery. Among the total cohort of 77 women, nearly half, 38 (49%), underwent unscheduled delivery most often due to bleeding (63%), followed by contractions (32%), and PPROM (5%).

The authors identified that for every episode of vaginal bleeding during pregnancy, the risk for unscheduled delivery increases by 3.8-fold, and more so in the setting of contractions and PPROM. Women who experienced antenatal bleeding delivered at a mean gestational age of 32.9 weeks (±3.3 weeks) and antenatal contractions at a mean of 33.3 weeks (± 2.9) (Figure 5.2).

Pri-Paz et al.[31] also showed that both a single episode and recurrent episodes of antenatal bleeding are associated with unscheduled delivery. Among a retrospective cohort of 48 women with placenta accreta, all of whom were suspected antenatally, 19/24 (79%) who underwent emergent delivery did so for bleeding versus 5/24 (21%) without bleeding ($p = 0.0005$).

Morbidity of Unscheduled Delivery

Cesarean Hysterectomy

The morbidities of cesarean hysterectomy for accreta are high, and early delivery is intended to avoid the added morbidities of emergent hysterectomy and suboptimal location. Early, scheduled delivery is advocated for maternal safety,[6,8,14–16] but what are the risks of unscheduled cesarean hysterectomy among women with suspected accreta? It is first important to consider the risks of cesarean hysterectomy.

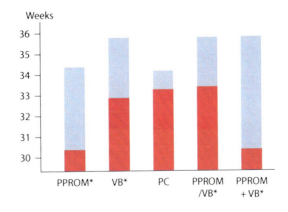

FIGURE 5.2 Decreasing gestational age at delivery in patients with placenta accreta and an additional risk factor for preterm delivery. The gestational age at delivery in patients with placenta accreta with an additional risk factor for preterm delivery absent is shown in red; the gestational age at delivery in patients with placenta accreta and an additional risk factor for preterm delivery is shown in black. PPROM = premature preterm rupture of membranes; VB = vaginal bleeding; PC = preterm contractions. *= *p*-value significant (0.001 or less). (Adapted from Bowman Z. et al. *Am J Obstet Gynecol,* 210, 241.e1–6, 2014.)

Compared to women undergoing nonobstetric hysterectomy, women undergoing peripartum hysterectomy have higher rates of bladder injury (9% vs. 1%), ureteral injury (0.7% vs. 0.1%), reoperation (4% vs. 0.5%), transfusion (46% vs. 4%), wound complications (10% vs. 3%), and venous thromboembolis (1% vs. 0.7%).[32] Women undergoing peripartum hysterectomy for placenta accreta had higher risks of complications compared to women undergoing peripartum hysterectomy for uterine atony, including more injuries to the bladder (OR 3.61), ureters (OR 2.87), and other organs (OR 2.01).[32] These differences are likely explained by distortions of anatomy, loss of tissue planes, friable tissue, and neovascularization with placenta accreta.[33] Cesarean hysterectomy in general is complicated by postoperative fever (11%), ileus (5.6%), and, in less than 3% of cases, bowel injury, vaginal cuff abscess, wound dehiscence, deep vein thrombosis, septic pelvic thrombophlebitis, and maternal death (Figure 5.3).[34,35]

Cesarean Hysterectomy with Placenta Percreta

Placenta percreta is associated with additional morbidities, requiring even greater surgical expertise at delivery. Surgical management may require intentional cystotomy to resect invaded bladder tissue and facilitate lateralization of the ureters.[36] The risk of cystotomy has been reported at 38%–50% with placenta percreta compared to 14%–18% with placenta accreta or increta.[37,38] Placenta percreta is also associated with increased risk of uterine rupture.[6]

It is reasonable to hypothesize that placenta increta/percreta is more likely to cause massive hemorrhage due to increasing invasiveness. The invading placental trophoblastic tissue lies closer to wide myometrial arteriovenous shunts rather than the smaller spiral arteries typical of trophoblastic implantation.[7,39] However, placenta increta/percreta is also more likely to be diagnosed antenatally and benefit from predelivery planning.

Morbidity of Emergent Cesarean Hysterectomy

Planned cesarean hysterectomy is generally thought to have less morbidity than emergent cesarean hysterectomy. Women undergoing emergent cesarean hysterectomy typically experience more blood loss, transfused units of blood, postoperative complications, and ICU admissions than women who undergo planned cesarean hysterectomy.[40] Higher rates of depression and posttraumatic stress disorder also occur.[41]

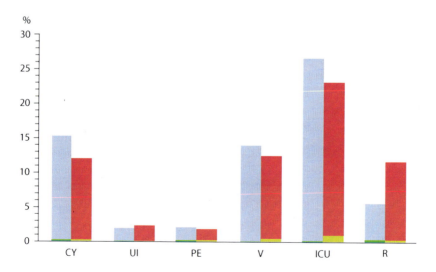

FIGURE 5.3 Increased morbidity of cesarean section in patients with placenta accreta or requiring hysterectomy. The percentage morbidity of patients without placenta accreta and with a risk factor is shown in green; the increased morbidity for patients with accreta is shown in blue. The percentage morbidity for patients without hysterectomy is shown in yellow; the increased morbidity for patients requiring cesarean hysterectomy with a risk factor is shown in red. Cy = cystotomy; UI = ureteral injury; PE = pulmonary embolus; V = ventilator; ICU = intensive care unit; R = reoperation. (Adapted from Silver RM et al., *Obstet Gynecol*, 107, 1226–1232, 2006.)

In a retrospective study of 76 cases of placenta accreta identified by International Classification of Disease, Ninth Edition (ICD-9) codes, 57 (75%) of the women who were suspected to have placenta accreta prior to delivery who underwent scheduled caesarean hysterectomy had a significantly lower mean blood loss (2.0 vs. 3.0 L, $p = 0.03$) compared with emergency delivery.[16] Eller et al. also consistently identified trends toward reduced morbidity in women with scheduled versus emergent cesarean hysterectomies.[16] Rates of ICU admission among the scheduled versus nonscheduled groups were 23% versus 31%, large volume blood transfusion was 32% versus 43%, ureteral injury was 5% versus 9%, intra-abdominal infection was 6% versus 9%, hospital readmission was 5% versus 18%, vesicovaginal fistula was 0% versus 6%, and early morbidity was 37% versus 57%. There was not a significant difference found based on scheduling in early morbidity (9[41%] scheduled vs. 16[46%] unscheduled, $p = 0.72$) or late morbidity (3[14%] scheduled vs. 8[23%] unscheduled, $p = 0.50$) among women with suspected placenta accreta, although numbers for some of these comparisons are small.[16]

In a retrospective cohort that included of 48 women identified through pathology records who were also suspected to have placenta accreta antenatally, ICU admission was more frequent among women who underwent emergent versus elective delivery.[31]

In contrast, when blood loss alone is considered, the impact of scheduled delivery is mixed. Pri-Paz et al.[31] found that, although women who experienced any antenatal bleeding were more likely to undergo emergent hysterectomy, during the emergent hysterectomy, EBL, and blood transfusion requirements did not differ when compared with women who underwent scheduled hysterectomy. Rac et al.[5] also found that EBL did not differ among women who delivered urgently for bleeding and those who underwent a scheduled delivery in a retrospective cohort where 60% of women had placenta accreta, 11% placenta increta, and 29% placenta percreta, not all of whom were suspected in advance.[5]

Centers of Excellence for Placenta Accreta

As described elsewhere in this book, women with placenta accreta who are cared for in a center of excellence are likely to experience less maternal hemorrhage and better outcomes.[42] A Center of Excellence (CoE) for placenta accreta should consist of at least a multidisciplinary team, an ICU and facilities, and blood services (Table 5.4).[42] It is important to consider that studies often do not report on available resources in the pertinent institution, further limiting some of the generalizability of data on timing of delivery and outcomes in accreta.

When a multidisciplinary approach was compared to management by a "standard" team in a nontertiary care center, the multidisciplinary approach was associated with a fivefold reduction in composite early maternal morbidity (OR 0.22, 95% confidence interval [CI] 0.07–0.70), less transfusion >4 units of packed red blood cells (43% vs. 61%, $p = 0.031$), and less reoperation within 7 days for bleeding (3% vs. 36%, $p < 0.001$).[43]

TABLE 5.4

Various Criteria for Placenta Accreta Centers of Excellence to Optimize Patient Outcomes

Multidisciplinary Team	Facilities	Transfusion Services
1. Maternal–fetal medicine physician or obstetrician	1. Interventional radiology	1. Massive transfusion capability
2. Pelvic surgeon (gynecologic oncology)	2. Surgical or medical intensive care unit	2. Cell saver and perfusionist
3. Obstetric anesthesiologist	3. Neonatal intensive care unit	3. Alternative blood products
4. Urologist		4. Transfusion medicine specialists or blood bank pathologists
5. Trauma surgeon		
6. Imaging experts		
7. Interventional radiologist		
8. Neonatologist		

Source: Adapted from Silver RM et al., *Am J Obstet Gynecol*, 212, 561–568, 2015. With permission.

Shamshirsaz et al. showed significant maternal benefits with a multidisciplinary approach with planned cesarean hysterectomy at 34–35 weeks, including less median EBL (2.1 L vs. 3.0 L, $p = 0.025$) and less need for emergency surgery (23% vs. 64%, $p = 0.001$)[33] In addition, a greater percentage of pregnancies in the multidisciplinary group received antenatal corticosteroids (60% vs. 39%, $p = 0.064$). In another study, Al-Khan et al. compared outcomes before and after implementation of a CoE type of approach. EBL, transfused packed red blood cells, and ICU admission were each reduced by 50% when delivery was planned at 34 weeks with a multidisciplinary team present.[7]

The presence of a gynecologic oncologist from the start of the procedure has been associated with a lower EBL and requirement for transfusion, despite the fact that such cases are more likely to involve placenta increta and percreta.[36] Cases where a gynecologic oncologist was called in emergently were associated with significantly more blood loss (4,400 mL vs. 1,800 mL).

Neonatal Morbidity

There are no prospective trials of delivery outcomes that assess neonatal morbidity based on delivery timing in women with suspected placenta accreta. Without such comparative studies, it is difficult to assess the magnitude of neonatal risk based on gestational age at delivery. Two existing comparative studies include cohorts where nearly all women underwent vaginal delivery and retained placenta was first identified at delivery.[44,45] Hence, these data cannot be used to guide delivery timing decisions for women with placenta previa with suspected accreta.

An ideal study would compare the risks of maternal and perinatal morbidity from maternal hemorrhage among women with suspected accreta to the risks of prematurity. Without such a study, fetal and neonatal risks must be extrapolated from what is known about fetal development and taken from existing studies that utilize nonideal comparison groups.

Iatrogenic Prematurity

About 30%–40% of preterm births are iatrogenic.[46,47] The increase in preterm deliveries has been associated with a decrease in stillbirth rate and decrease in the infant mortality rate.[46,48] These declines in morbidity and mortality were most pronounced at 34–36 weeks' gestation and larger among iatrogenic preterm births than among spontaneous preterm births (OR 0.75 vs. 0.82, $p < 0.001$), plausibly due to the cessation of risk posed by the maternal condition that delivery brings about.

Fetal/Neonatal Morbidity

The most frequent neonatal risk at 34 weeks is respiratory morbidity. Between 34 and 36 weeks' gestation, fetal lung tissue matures from terminal sacs dominated by Type 1 squamous epithelial cells to alveoli containing Type II surfactant producing cuboidal epithelial cells.[48]

The odds of respiratory distress/hyaline membrane disease decreases 40-fold between 34 and 39–40 weeks.[49] The risk is substantially decreased with each additional week of gestational age, with the risk decreasing 22-fold by 35 weeks, and with an additional 9-decrease by 36 weeks.[49]

In addition to respiratory distress, the risks of intraventricular hemorrhage, sepsis, necrotizing enterocolitis, and need for phototherapy are increased in later preterm infants compared to infants born at 39 weeks. When aggregated to include one or more of these morbidities, 34% of births at 34 weeks had morbidity, decreasing to 24% at 35 weeks, 17% at 36 weeks, and 14% at 37 weeks compared with the reference standard of 14% at 39 weeks.[50]

A systemic review of 22 studies totaling almost 30 million infants compared outcomes between late preterm (34 weeks 0/7 days' gestation to 36 weeks 6/7 days' gestation) and term infants (Table 5.5).[51]

Late preterm births are associated with increased risk of RDS (relative risk [RR] 17.3), need for mechanical ventilation or intubation (RR 4.9), any intraventricular hemorrhage (RR 4.9), necrotizing enterocolitis (RR 7.5), and neonatal death (RR 5.9). Long-term adverse outcomes include significantly increased risks of cerebral palsy (RR 3.1), mental retardation (RR 1.5), schizophrenia (RR 1.4), developmental delay/disability (RR 1.4), and infant death in the first year after delivery (RR 3.7). Some of these risks may be due to the pregnancy complication necessitating preterm delivery rather than to prematurity itself.[51]

Perinatal Morbidity of Placenta Accreta

As mentioned, two studies have been conducted among women with clinical sequalae consistent with retained placenta at delivery, most frequently following vaginal delivery, with cesarean rates of only 4.8%[45] and 11.3%.[44] Among women with any form of retained placenta, there were increased rates of low birthweight, APGAR scores <7, and total perinatal mortality (6.7%).[44] Newborns of women with retained placenta had a fivefold increase in small for gestational age or weight less than the 10th percentile (Table 5.6).[45]

In a population-based study of morbidly adherent placenta that used *ICD-10* discharge codes from Ireland, the rate of stillbirth among women with the condition was increased 4.7-fold (95% CI 2.4–9.1).[52]

Among women with suspected placenta accreta and planned delivery at 34–35 weeks, the rate of preterm birth (by definition) is 100%. In a systematic review and meta-analysis of observational and experimental studies of women with placenta accreta, many in which the diagnosis of accreta was retrospective, the rate of preterm delivery was 57.7%.[53] Bailit et al. observed that when morbidly adherent placenta was suspected before delivery, newborns were delivered at early gestational ages (35.6 weeks [33.6–36.9] suspected vs. 37.8 weeks [35.4–39.9] not suspected, $p < 0.001$), were more likely to require ventilator support (24 [28.6% (95% CI 18.9–38.2)] suspected vs. 8 [10.8% (95% CI 3.7–17.9), p = 0.006]), and were more likely to be admitted to the neonatal intensive care unit (55 [65.5% (95% CI 55.3–75.6)] suspected vs. 25 [33.8% (95% CI 23.0–44.6), p < 0.001]).[11]

Planned cesarean delivery is a risk factor for respiratory morbidity independent of prematurity; the incidence of respiratory morbidity is significantly higher for the group delivered by caesarean section before the onset of labor (35.5/1,000) compared with vaginal delivery (5.3/1,000) (OR 6.8; 95% CI 5.2–8.9).[54]

Another factor to consider is whether the patient received corticosteroids, which decrease the risk of severe neonatal respiratory morbidity. They should be administered 48 hours prior to delivery in order to have an optimal effect. Thus, cases of antenatally diagnosed accreta with scheduled delivery are more likely to receive steroids than undiagnosed cases. Available studies on accreta have not stratified analyses based on whether patients received steroids.

TABLE 5.5

Neonatal Outcomes of Late Preterm Births

Short-Term Outcome	Weeks Gestational Age, AR% (RR)			
	34 weeks	35 weeks	36 weeks	Full Term
Neonatal mortality	0.57 (10.1)	0.34 (6.3)	0.23 (3.9)	0.06
5-Minute APGAR <3	0.14 (2.1)	0.18 (2.7)	0.09 (1.3)	0.07
Intubation or mechanical ventilation	3.6 (12.4)	1.7 (5.3)	0.79 (2.8)	0.26
Nasal CPAP	8.8 (25.9)	5.3 (16.4)	2.1	0.26
TTN	5.1 (15.4)	3.3 (9.6)	2.0 (5.7)	0.35
RDS	10.6 (48.4)	6.0 (28.6)	2.7 (10.9)	0.36
NEC	0.21 (11.7)	0.06 (7.1)	0.02 (2.5)	<0.01
IVH (grade I–IV)	0.46 (19.5)	0.22 (9.4)	0.08 (3.3)	0.02
Feeding problems	51.0 (9.6)	34.0 (6.4)	22.0 (4.1)	5.3
Hyperbilirubinemia	42.9 (16.1)	16.0 (6.0)	16.0 (6.0)	2.7
Jaundice requiring phototherapy	10.3 (10.6)	6.0 (6.7)	2.4 (2.0)	1.3

Abbreviations: AR, absolute risk; CPAP, continuous positive airway pressure; IVH, intraventricular hemorrhage; NEC, necrotizing enterocolitis; RDS, respiratory distress syndrome; RR, relative risk; TTN, transient tachypnea of newborn.

TABLE 5.6

Various Neonatal Outcomes for Placenta Accreta
and Placenta Previa

Neonatal Outcome	Risk Ratio or Difference of Outcome
Accreta Present	
Gestational age at delivery	1.5 weeks earlier
Birth weight	Weigh 240 g less at birth
Previa Present	
Preterm delivery	5.32 increased risk
Neonatal death	5.44 increased risk
NICU admission	4.09 increased risk

Abbreviation: NICU, neonatal intensive care unit.

Delivery Timing in Practice

Three surveys of members of the SMFM[4,55] and the American College of Obstetricians and Gynecologists (ACOG)[56] suggest that in practice, many US maternal–fetal medicine (MFM) specialists and obstetricians recommend delivery later than 34–35 weeks. It should be noted, however, that these surveys were completed[4,55] or initially sent to respondents[56] prior to the publication of the recommendation by the NICHD for delivery at 34–35 weeks among women with suspected accreta.[3]

Esakoff et al.[4] surveyed members of SMFM by mail, between 6/2009 and 9/2009, regarding management practices for women with suspected placenta accreta. The response rate was low at 19.4%. The authors found that most providers recommend delivery of women with suspected accreta at 36 weeks or beyond, with differences in recommendations based on years in practice and geographic region. Approximately, 50% of physicians in practice for ≥20 years recommended delivery at 36 weeks, whereas physicians in practice for >20 years were divided between a recommendation for delivery at 36 weeks (35%) and 38 weeks (34%), $p = 0.001$. Physicians in the Northwest were the most likely to deliver at 35 weeks (17%) versus 2%–4% in other regions ($p < 0.003$).

In a similar survey of members of SMFM, Jolley et al.[55] found that 48.4% of SMFM members scheduled women with suspected accreta for delivery at 36 weeks. The authors conducted a web-based survey prior to the publication of the NICHD recommendation, with a 29% response rate. Forty-eight percent of respondents reported delivering asymptomatic women with high suspicion for accreta at 36 weeks. Only 4.4% of respondents recommended delivery of such women at 34 weeks, 5.3% at 35 weeks, 28.4% at 37 weeks, 7.3% at 38 weeks, and 5.7% at 39 weeks.

In a mailed survey of members of ACOG, with a 51.1% response rate of whom 85% were general obstetrician/gynecologists, most (38.8%) recommended delivery at 36 weeks.[56] Of note, the first surveys were mailed 1 month prior to the publication of the NICHD recommendations, with three subsequent mailings to nonresponders sent afterward. Data are not shown regarding responses stratified by timing of return of the survey. Only 2.4% of respondents recommended scheduled delivery at 34 weeks, 34.3% at 38 weeks, and disturbingly, 18.1% recommended delivery at term unless the patient went into labor.

Conclusion

Existing studies have helped identify women at risk for emergent delivery in the setting of suspected accreta—very short cervix, contractions, vaginal bleeding, and PPROM—and no studies have identified women not at risk for emergent delivery.

Until there are convincing data for prolongation of pregnancy among women with placenta previa and suspected accreta, the risks of potential morbidity of uncontrolled bleeding seem to support current NICHD recommendations for delivery at 34–35 weeks and 6 days.

REFERENCES

1. Wu S, Kocherginsky M, Hibbard J. Abnormal placentation: Twenty-year analysis. *Am J Obstet Gynecol.* 2005;192:1458–1461.
2. Mogos MF, Salemi JL, Ashley M, Whiteman VE, Salihu HM. Recent trends in placenta accreta in the United States and its impact on maternal-fetal morbidity and healthcare-associated costs, 1998–2011. *J Matern Fetal Neonatal Med.* 2016;29:1077–1082.
3. Spong CY, Mercer BM, D'alton M et al. Timing of indicated late-preterm and early-term birth. *Obstet Gynecol.* 2011;118:323–233.
4. Esakoff TF, Handler SJ, Granados JM et al. PAMUS: Placenta accreta management across the United States. *J Matern Fetal Neonatal Med.* 2012;25:761–765.
5. Rac MW, Wells CE, Twickler DM et al. Placenta accreta and vaginal bleeding according to gestational age at delivery. *Obstet Gynecol.* 2015;125:808–813.
6. O'Brien J, Barton J, Donaldson E. The management of placenta percreta: Conservative and operative strategies. *Am J Obstet Gynecol.* 1996;175:1632–1638.
7. Al-Khan A, Gupta V, Illsley N et al. Maternal and fetal outcomes in placenta accreta after institution of team-managed care. *Reprod Sci.* 2014;21:761–771.
8. Robinson B, Grobman W. Effectiveness of timing strategies for delivery of individuals with placenta previa and accreta. *Obstet Gynecol.* 2010;116:835–842.
9. Belfort M. Placenta accreta. *Am J Obstet Gynecol.* 2010;203:430–439.
10. Ekin A, Gezer C, Solmaz U et al. Predictors of severity in primary postpartum hemorrhage. *Arch Gynecol Obstet.* 2015;292:1247–154.
11. Bailit J, Grobman W, Rice M et al. Morbidly adherent placenta treatments and outcomes. *Obstet Gynecol.* 2015;125:683–689.
12. Wright J, Pri-Paz S, Herzog T et al. Predictors of massive blood loss in women with placenta accreta. *Am J Obstet Gynecol.* 2011;205:38.e1–6.
13. Stotler B, Padmanabhan A, Devine P et al. Transfusion requirements in obstetric patients with placenta accreta. *Transfusion.* 2011;51:2627–2633.
14. Warshak CR, Ramos GA, Eskander R et al. Effect of predelivery diagnosis in 99 consecutive cases of placenta accreta. *Obstet Gynecol.* 2010;115:65–69.
15. Oyelese Y, Smulian J. Placenta previa, placenta accreta, and vasa previa. *Obstet Gynecol.* 2006;107:927–941.
16. Eller A, Porter T, Soisson P et al. Optimal management strategies for placenta accreta. *BJOG.* 2009;116:648–654.
17. Zlatnik M, Cheng Y, Norton M et al. Placenta previa and the risk of preterm delivery. *J Matern Fetal Neonatal Med.* 2007;20:719–723.
18. Zlatnik M, Little S, Kohli P et al. When should women with placenta previa be delivered? A decision analysis. *J Reprod Med.* 2010;55:373–381.
19. Bowman Z, Manuck T; Eller A et al. Risk factors for unscheduled delivery in patients with placenta accreta. *Am J Obstet Gynecol.* 2014;210:241. e1–6.
20. Meller C, Izbizky G, Otaño L. Timing of delivery in placenta accreta. *Am J Obstet Gynecol.* 2014 Oct;211(4):438–439.
21. Stafford I, Dashe J, Shivvers S et al. Ultrasonographic cervical length and risk of hemorrhage in pregnancies with placenta previa. *Obstet Gynecol.* 2010;116:595–600.
22. Ghi T, Contro E, Martina T et al. Cervical length and risk of antepartum bleeding in women with complete placenta previa. *Ultrasound Obstet Gynecol.* 2009;33:209–212.
23. Sekiguchi A, Nakai A, Okuda N et al. Consecutive cervical length measurements as a predictor of preterm cesarean section in complete placenta previa. *J Clin Ultrasound.* 2015;43:17–22.
24. Zaitoun M, El Behery M, Abd El Hameed A et al. Does cervical length and the lower placental edge thickness measurement correlates with clinical outcome in cases of complete placenta previa? *Arch Gynecol Obstet.* 2011;284:867–873.
25. Fukushima K, Fujiwara A, Anami A et al. Cervical length predicts placental adherence and massive hemorrhage in placenta previa. *J Obstet Gynaecol Res.* 2012;38:192–197.
26. Polat M, Kahramanoglu I, Senol T et al. Shorter the cervix, more difficult the placenta percreta operations. *J Matern Fetal Neonatal Med.* 2015;15:1–5.

27. Tikkanen M, Paavonen J, Loukovaara M et al. Antenatal diagnosis of placenta accreta leads to reduced blood loss. *Acta Obstet Gynecol Scand.* 2011;90:1140–1146.
28. Thurn L, Lindqvist PG, Jakobsson M et al. Abnormally invasive placenta-prevalence, risk factors and antenatal suspicion: Results from a large population-based pregnancy cohort study in the Nordic countries. *BJOG.* 2015;123:1348–1355. DOI: 10.1111/1471-0528.13547
29. Grace Tan S, Jobling T, Wallace E et al. Surgical management of placenta accreta: A 10-year experience. *Acta Obstet Gynecol Scand.* 2013;92:445–450.
30. Fitzpatrick K, Sellers S, Spark P et al. The management and outcomes of placenta accreta, increta, and percreta in the UK: A population-based descriptive study. *BJOG.* 2014;121:62–71.
31. Pri-Paz S, Fuchs K, Gaddipati S et al. Comparison between emergent and elective delivery in women with placenta accreta. *J Matern Fetal Neonatal Med.* 2013;26:1007–1011.
32. Wright J, Devine P, Shah M et al. Morbidity and mortality of peripartum hysterectomy. *Obstet Gynecol.* 2010;115:1187–1193.
33. Shamshirsaz A, Fox K, Salmanian B et al. Maternal morbidity in patients with morbidly adherent placent atreated with and without a standardized multidisciplinary approach. *Am J Obstet Gynecol.* 2015;212:218.e1–9.
34. Shellhaas C, Gilbert S, Landon M et al. The frequency and complication rates of hysterectomy accompanying cesarean delivery. *Obstet Gynecol.* 2009;114:224–229.
35. Silver RM, Landon MB, Rouse DJ et al.; National Institute of Child Health and Human Development Maternal-Fetal Medicine Units Network. Maternal morbidity associated with multiple repeat cesarean deliveries. *Obstet Gynecol.* 2006 Jun;107(6):1226–1232.
36. Brennan D, Schulze B, Chetty N et al. Surgical management of abnormally invasive placenta: a retrospective cohort study demonstrating the benefits of a standardized operative approach. *Acta Obstet Gynecol Scand.* 2015;94:1380–1386.
37. Brookfield K, Goodnough L, Lyell D et al. Perioperative and transfusion outcomes in women undergoing cesarean hysterectomy for abnormal placentation. *Transfusion.* 2014;54:1530–1536.
38. Woldu S, Ordonez M, Devine P et al. Urologic considerations of placenta accreta: A contemporary tertiary care institutional experience. *Urol Int.* 2014;93:74–79.
39. Chantraine F, Blacher S, Berndt S et al. Abnormal vascular architecture at the placental-maternal interface in placenta increta. *Am J Obstet Gynecol.* 2012;207:188.e1–9.
40. Briery C, Rose C, Hudson W et al. Planned vs emergent cesarean hysterectomy. *Am J Obstet Gynecol.* 2007;197:154. e1–5.
41. de la Cruz C, Coulter M, O'Rourke K et al. Post-traumatic stress disorder following emergency peripartum hysterectomy. *Arch Gynecol Obstet.* 2016;294:681–688. DOI:10.1007/s00404-016-4008-y
42. Silver RM, Fox K, Barton J et al. Center of excellence for placenta accreta. *Am J Obstet Gynecol.* 2015;212:561–568.
43. Eller A, Bennett M, Sharshiner M et al. Maternal morbidity in cases of placenta accreta managed by a multidisciplinary care team compared with standard obstetric care. *Obstet Gynecol.* 2011;117:331–337.
44. Vinograd A, Wainstock T, Mazor M et al. Placenta accreta is an independent risk factor for late pre-term birth and perinatal mortality. *J Matern Fetal Neonatal Med.* 2015;28:1381–1387.
45. Gielchinsky Y, Mankuta D, Rojansky N et al. Perinatal outcome of pregnancies complicated by placenta accreta. *Obstet Gynecol.* 2004;104:527–530.
46. Joseph K, Demissie K, Kramer M. Obstetric intervention, stillbirth, and preterm birth. *Semin Perinatol.* 2002;26:250–259.
47. Wong A, Grobman W. Medically indicated—Iatrogenic prematurity. *Clin Perinatol.* 2011;38:423–439.
48. Mahoney A, Jain L. Respiratory disorders in moderately preterm, late preterm, and early term infants. *Clin Perinatol.* 2013;40:665–678.
49. Hibbard J, Wilkins I, Sun L et al. Respiratory morbidity in late preterm births. *JAMA.* 2010 Jul 28;304:419–425.
50. McIntire D, Leveno K. Neonatal mortality and morbidity rates in late preterm births compared with births at term. *Obstet Gynecol.* 2008;111:35–41.
51. Teune M, Bakhuizen S, Gyamfi Bannerman C et al. A systematic review of severe morbidity in infants born late preterm. *Am J Obstet Gynecol.* 2011;205:374.e1–9.
52. Upson K, Silver RM, Greene R et al. Placenta accreta and maternal morbidity in the Republic of Ireland, 2005–2010. *J Matern Fetal Neonatal Med.* 2014;27:24–29.

53. Vahanian S, Lavery J, Ananth C et al. Placental implantation abnormalities and risk of preterm delivery: A systematic review and metaanalysis. *Am J Obstet Gynecol.* 2015;213:S78–90.
54. Ryan C, Hughes P. Neonatal respiratory morbidity and mode of delivery at term: Influence of timing of elective caesarean section. *Br J Obstet Gynaecol.* 1995;102:843–844.
55. Jolley J, Nageotte M, Wing D et al. Management of placenta accreta: A survey of maternal-fetal medicine practitioners. *J Matern Fetal Neonatal Med.* 2012;25:756–760.
56. Wright J, Silver RM, Bonanno C et al. Practice patterns and knowledge of obstetricians and gynecologists regarding placenta accreta. *J Matern Fetal Neonatal Med.* 2013;26:1602–1609.

6

Surgical Management of Placenta Accreta

William M. Burke, Annette Perez-Delboy, and Jason D. Wright

CONTENTS

Introduction

In the United States, it is estimated that peripartum hysterectomies are performed in approximately 0.08% of all deliveries.[1] Traditionally, the most common indication for this procedure has been obstetric hemorrhage due to uterine atony. A large study from the United Kingdom noted that more than half of peripartum hysterectomies were performed for uterine atony and 38% were a result of placenta accreta.[2] More recently, population-based analyses demonstrate that abnormal placentation is the indication for the majority of peripartum hysterectomies.[3] A majority of women with morbidly adherent placenta require surgical management at some point in their course. While there is debate about the optimal surgical management of women with placenta accreta, regardless of the strategy chosen, treatment is associated with substantial morbidity and mortality. In this chapter, we discuss the surgical management of morbidly adherent placenta in a variety of scenarios. For all scenarios, accurate and early diagnosis, preoperative planning and preparation, and the involvement of a multidisciplinary team are the key factors in optimizing outcomes.[4]

Preoperative Preparation

The management of placenta accreta involves careful preoperative planning and preparation to minimize the morbidity and mortality. Prior to the planned surgical procedure, a number of secondary measures can be undertaken that may reduce perioperative morbidity. One of the primary goals is to put in place a multidisciplinary team to facilitate a coordinated delivery.[4] The multidisciplinary team often includes obstetricians, gynecologic oncologists, anesthesiologists, urologists, vascular surgeons, pediatricians, critical care medicine specialists, and nurses. Use of a dedicated, multidisciplinary team has been associated with improved outcomes.[5] Preoperative team meetings with review of imaging findings and operative planning may help optimize outcomes. Women with suspected placenta accreta are at substantial risk for preterm delivery due to bleeding and other complications. Several reports show that outcomes are worse and morbidity is higher in women who deliver emergently or in an unplanned fashion.[6–9] Given these findings, many experts support a scheduled, preterm delivery so the operative procedure can be undertaken in a controlled and optimal fashion.

Development of a Multidisciplinary Team

The most crucial component of the antepartum management of placenta accreta is the establishment of a multidisciplinary team that will discuss the case prior to delivery (Table 6.1).[4] The team should include all service lines that may be involved in management during the antenatal and postnatal periods. It may be helpful to create a contact list that includes team members who can be utilized to notify appropriate staff of updates and delivery dates. Further, the contact list is useful during emergent scenarios. Many referral centers have created institutional guidelines, flow charts, and check lists to ensure that each case is managed using a standardized approach. There is evidence that patients managed by a multidisciplinary care team are less likely to require large-volume blood transfusion, reoperation within 7 days of delivery for bleeding complications, and to experience prolonged maternal admission to the intensive care unit (ICU) than women managed by standard obstetric care.[7]

Preoperative Imaging

The main screening modality for abnormal placentation is ultrasound imaging. Patients should undergo transabdominal and transvaginal ultrasound evaluation of the placenta including documentation of placental position and location. Using the diagnostic criteria for abnormal placentation as Finberg et al. first described in 1992,[10] the sonogram should specifically look for evidence of lacunar spaces, the absence of a retroplacental hypoechoic space, and irregular interface between the placenta and myometrium. Color flow mapping may demonstrate a lack of normal myometrial–placental interface in the myometrium. Other sonographic findings that may improve the detection of placentas accreta include the myometrial thinning to <1 mm, extension of villi beyond the myometrium to the serosa or bladder, and an increase

TABLE 6.1

Multidisciplinary Team for the Management of Placenta Accreta

Surgical Team	Ancillary Services
Maternal–fetal medicine	Blood bank
Gynecologic oncology/surgery	Perfusion services
Obstetric anesthesiology	Obstetric nursing
Urology	Surgical intensive care unit
Interventional radiology	Neonatal intensive care unit and pediatrics
Vascular surgery	Operating room staff
Trauma surgery	Radiology

in vascularity between the uterine and bladder wall with turbulent color flow identified on Doppler ultrasound.[11] Pilloni et al. used a two criteria system to increase the sensitivity and specificity of the diagnosis of placenta accreta. The diagnosis was based on the identification of at least two of the following characteristics: (1) loss or irregularity of the hypoechoic area between the uterus and placenta, the "retroplacental clear zone," (2) thinning or interruption of the uterine serosa–bladder wall interface, (3) myometrial thickness <1 mm, (4) turbulent placental lacunae with high velocity flow (>15 cm/s), (5) increased vascularity of the uterine serosa–bladder wall interface, and (6) loss of the vascular arch parallel to the basal plate and irregular intraplacental vascularization.[12] While these characteristics are predictive of placenta accreta, studies have noted that there is significant interobserver variability in the interpretation of sonograms for placenta accreta.[13]

Pelvic magnetic resonance imaging (MRI) may be performed as an adjuvant to sonography when the placenta is difficult to visualize because of increased body mass index or a posterior placenta.[14] MRI also provides greater soft tissue contrast and a larger field of view than ultrasonography, which may be helpful in diagnosing cases of abnormal placentation with equivocal ultrasound findings. Lax et al. were the first to study features associated with placental invasion on prenatal MRI.[15] MRI findings associated with abnormal placentation were abnormal bulging of the lower uterine segment, heterogeneity of signal intensity, and dark intraplacental bands.[16,17] These features may be especially important in posterior placental implantation.[14] Images should be reviewed by the multidisciplinary team to confirm the diagnosis, assess the degree of abnormal placentation, and guide management.

Preoperative Anemia

All patients should be screened for anemia at the initial obstetric visit, 28 weeks gestation, and at any time of admission. The aim is to maintain a hematocrit above 30 g/dL with routine supplementation of iron and folic acid to achieve this goal. A relatively higher hemoglobin and erythrocyte level preoperatively is associated with decreased transfusion requirements. If anemia is identified, a complete laboratory evaluation is initiated to better define the etiology of the anemia. The two most common causes of anemia in pregnancy are iron deficiency and acute blood loss. Iron requirements increase during pregnancy due to a failure to maintain sufficient levels of iron. Iron deficiency anemia is defined as a ferritin level of less than 10–15 µg. Unless a contraindication exists, patients should be initiated on oral iron and folic acid therapy. Parenteral iron therapy is considered for those patients with iron deficiency anemia who cannot tolerate or are noncompliant with oral therapy. Erythropoietin stimulating agents should be considered for patients with severe (hemoglobin <8 g/dL) or persistent anemia (Table 6.2). If erythropoietin stimulating agents or intravenous iron is considered, hematology consultation is essential for a full evaluation.

Hospital systems that support early recognition and a rapid, coordinated response to extreme blood loss can limit maternal morbidity and improve maternal survival. Obstetric hemorrhage emergencies should be handled with the same level of urgency and preparation as a cardiac code. Any team member

TABLE 6.2

Management of Anemia in Women with Suspected Abnormalities of Placentation

Oral Therapy	Parenteral Therapy
Ferrous sulfate 325 mg qd-tid	Iron sucrose formulation 20 mg iron per mL
Ascorbic acid (vitamin C) 500 mg with every dose of iron	Iron sucrose (Venofer) 100 mg IV 1–2 times per week
Folic acid 400 mcg qd	Erythropoietin stimulating agents
	• Epogen 600 units/kg q week, maximum dose of 40,000 units/week
	• Increase to 60,000 units per week if no response after 2 weeks
	• Confirm adequate iron stores
Alternative formulations of elemental iron	
• Fe fumarate 200–300 mg bid-tid	

can call for help and activate a maternal hemorrhage response as clinically indicated. Massive transfusion protocols (MTP) involve the early utilization of blood products and ensure rapid availability of transfusion products for patients with suspected massive hemorrhage. In order to optimize patient care and safety, communication with the blood bank to develop new strategies and guidelines to facilitate the timely availability of blood components is paramount. Adequate blood products should be available at the time of delivery for scheduled placenta accretas. At our institution, we typically prepare 20 units of packed red blood cells (PRBCs), 20 units of fresh-frozen plasma (FFP), two six-packs of platelets, and 10 units of cryoprecipitate. Follow-up communication is made to determine the efficacy of the released products and the need for additional products. Communication with blood bank personnel as well as optimizing transfusion protocols in order to be able to order a massive transfusion at the time of peripartum hysterectomy may improve outcome.[18] Protocols and procedures for blood acquisitions and administration are essential in the success of the case.

Acute normovolemic hemodilution can be used safely in the pregnant woman at high risk for excessive intraoperative blood loss.[19] Hemodilution is performed before starting the case by collection of two to three units of whole blood and replacing it with crystalloid. In order to be a candidate, the patient should have a baseline hemoglobin of 10 g/dL, no history of cardiac disease, and a predicted blood loss of less than 20% of the patient's volume.

Autologous donation is safe to offer during pregnancy. Most patients have a starting hematocrit of at least 34% and donate between one and three units of blood. Each donation is given about 1 week apart and the last should be at least 2 weeks prior to delivery.[20] The patient with placenta accreta can rarely produce enough autologous blood to avoid homologous blood transfusion. This process may be practical for patients with unusual antibodies.

Preoperative Counseling

Physicians concerns for a placenta accreta should be heightened if the patient has had an invasive procedure on the uterus or uterine cavity. Major risk factors include placenta previa, prior cesarean delivery, myomectomy, dilation and curettage, endometrial ablation, and Asherman's syndrome. Women with suspicious imaging findings should be counseled about the risks of preterm delivery, hysterectomy, and obstetric hemorrhage, and care should be tailored to their individual needs and wishes. Preoperative counseling should also include a review of operative risks including intraoperative injury.

The patient should understand that there is a substantial risk for injury to the genitourinary tract during these procedures.[6,7] Cystotomy and ureteral injury are relatively common. Cystotomy is required in approximately 15% of cases.[21] Ureteral identification can be difficult, particularly if the placenta invades into the parametrium. The rate of ureteral injury is 2%–6% but can be reduced when ureteral stents are placed for identification and protection of ureters.[6,22] It is part of our standard treatment to perform cystoscopy to evaluate the bladder for possible placental invasion and place ureteral stents electively in these patients. Although ureteral stents do not always prevent ureteral injury, it makes them easier to recognize in an emergency.

Bleeding at the time of peripartum hysterectomy for placenta accreta is often substantial.[2,8,23] As such, preoperative preparedness for massive transfusion is essential. Nearly 90% of patients require blood products,[24] while 38% of patients need a massive blood transfusion (>20 units of red cells). Fevers and infectious morbidity appears to be the most common complication and occurs in up to one-third of women.[25]

There is a 30% risk of an ICU admission, thromboembolic disease, readmission, reoperation, poor wound healing, and a reported rate of surgical re-exploration ranging from 4% to 33%. The utilization of intensive care is variable, while up to 13% of women require continued mechanical ventilation. The risk of maternal death should also be discussed, since it is reported to be as high as 7% (although less in most recent series)[2,21,22] with a median length of hospital stay after peripartum hysterectomy of 4–5 days.[1,25]

Preoperative counseling should also include a discussion of bilateral tubal ligation in the event that hysterectomy is not necessary at the time of delivery. Future pregnancy should be avoided when possible, as it will be associated with an increased risk of placental invasion and maternal risk. Women managed in the outpatient setting should be counseled that bleeding, contractions, or pain should prompt immediate return to the hospital for evaluation. Women should have someone readily available in case this situation arises and have immediate access to the hospital.

Inpatient Observation

All patients are admitted prior to the day of scheduled delivery to facilitate preoperative preparation and finalize planning. Earlier admissions in the pregnancy recommended if there is vaginal bleeding during the second or third trimester, preterm labor, cervical shortening, or in patients who live an extended distance from the hospital or are unattended at home. Patients with placenta previa and a cervical length of 30 mm or less at 32 weeks have an increased risk of hemorrhage, uterine activity, and preterm birth.[26]

Delivery Planning

The optimal time for delivery is unclear, but given the increased likelihood for hysterectomy, hemorrhage, transfusion, complications, and possible maternal death, many experts recommend preterm delivery so that the operative procedure can be undertaken in a controlled fashion. Timing of delivery may have a crucial impact on maternal and perinatal outcome. O'Brien et al. reported that after 35 weeks, 93% of patients with placenta accreta experience hemorrhage necessitating delivery.[22] To avoid an emergency cesarean on the one hand and to minimize complications of prematurity on the other, it is acceptable to schedule cesarean at 34–35 weeks without confirmation of fetal lung maturity.[27] Warshak et al. reported that planned delivery at 34–35 weeks of gestation in a cohort of 99 cases of accreta did not significantly increase neonatal morbidity.[28] One decision analysis found that a scheduled delivery at 34 weeks of gestation was the preferred strategy to balance maternal and neonatal morbidity.[29] The patient and obstetrician must weigh risks of neonatal prematurity and the benefit of a planned delivery before the onset of labor. However, patients with a prenatal diagnosis of placenta accreta should be delivered no later than 36–37 weeks gestation. This might be appropriate for those patients who have remained stable with no vaginal bleeding or preterm labor and have an obstetrical history of a term delivery. Women who are asymptomatic with a lower clinical suspicion of an accreta and no previa should be delivered closer to term.

In our institution, steroids are administered to improve neonatal outcome for any patient at risk for delivery prior to 37 weeks gestation, recurrent vaginal bleeding, or placenta percreta.[30] All cases with heightened suspicion for accreta on preoperative imaging will be delivered in the main operating rooms. The American College of Obstetrics and Gynecology (ACOG) committee opinion on placenta accreta indicates that delivery timing should be individualized based on the antenatal suspicion of abnormal placentation, degree of invasion, surgical risks, maternal status, and obstetric history.

Delivery Day

On the day of the scheduled delivery, a preoperative checklist (Figure 6.1) should be utilized to prepare the operating room and team. After induction of anesthesia, vascular catheters (embolization and balloon occlusion) can be placed. A staff member from institutional research (IR) or vascular should be readily available until completion of the surgery for management of the catheters. Blood products for possible massive transfusion should available in the operating room before starting the case. Cell saver technology and credentialed staff should be immediately available in the operating room prior to initiating the delivery. A neonatology team composed of a physician, nurses, and/or respiratory therapists should be present at all deliveries and a checklist to ensure preparedness for delivery should be used.

Accreta Team Checklist

Morgan Stanley
**Children's Hospital
of NewYork-Presbyterian**
Columbia University Medical Center

Complete the checklist by indicating Y (Yes) or N (No)

DATE: _____ TIME: _____

ACTIVITY		✔		
		Y	N	N/A
Maternal Fetal Medicine				
GYN Oncology				
OB Anesthesia				
Urology				
Interventional Radiology				
Vascular Surgery				
Cardiothoracic Surgery				
NICU				
Main OR Scheduling				
Nursing / Scrubs				
Blood Bank				
Cell Saver				
SICU				

FIGURE 6.1 Accreta team checklist. (Courtesy of Columbia University Medical Center.)

Surgical Management of Expected Placenta Accreta

Placenta accreta is one of the most common reasons for cesarean hysterectomy. In a population-based descriptive study using the UK Obstetric Surveillance System, Knight reported that 38% of peripartum hysterectomies were due to morbidly adherent placenta.[2] With early recognition and planned surgical intervention, the morbidity associated with this procedure can be reduced, especially when compared to emergent delivery due to unexpected obstetrical hemorrhage.[7,28] Data also indicate improved outcomes when women diagnosed with placenta accreta are cared for at high-volume, tertiary centers compared to facilities that care for few women with morbidly adherent placenta disease.[5,31]

Preoperative planning is essential when placental abnormalities are suspected. A review of available imaging including MRI and ultrasound will facilitate surgical planning. It should be recognized that available imaging modalities are often inaccurate in defining the extent of placental invasion in women with placenta accreta. Prior to proceeding to the operating room, the possibility of hysterectomy and the morbidity of the procedure should be discussed with patients and informed consent obtained. Preoperative preparation, as outlined previously in this chapter, should include a discussion of the proposed surgery, placement of internal iliac catheters by interventional radiology or vascular surgery, retrograde ureteral stent placement by urology, initiation of massive blood transfusion protocol, activation of cell saver and perfusion staff, ICU notification, and mobilization of experienced surgical nursing and technician teams.

Once the patient is ready for the surgery to begin, it is essential to ensure proper patient positioning and the availability of all necessary surgical equipment. Strong consideration should be given to placing all patients with suspected accreta in lithotomy position to allow access to the vagina. Though there is some controversy as to which surgical incision should be used, a vertical midline incision is typically utilized to obtain maximal exposure, facilitate delivery of the gravid uterus, and allow exploration of the upper abdomen, pelvic sidewalls, and retroperitoneum. Although a midline incision provides optimal exposure, a Maylard or Cherney incision can also be considered.

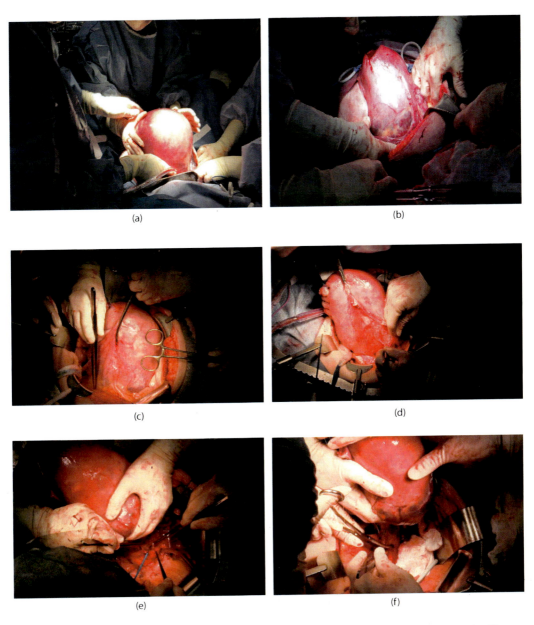

FIGURE 6.2   (a) Uterus with placenta accreta exteriorized prior to hysterotomy. (b) Uterus placed under traction. Placenta accreta with increased vascularity bulging into the lower uterine segment and left parametrium. (c) Dissection of the placenta from the surrounding soft tissue. (d) Uterus further mobilized and placenta being dissected away from the bladder. The retroperitoneal space has been opened. (e) Continuation of the dissection of the placenta away from the bladder. The dissection has been carried below the placenta which is shown protected by the surgeon's hand. Perforating vessels are cauterized. (f) The dissection has now been carried down to below the area of placental invasion. The uterus with the placenta is elevated and a relatively normal lower uterine segment is visible.

After gaining access to the abdomen, the uterus should be inspected to confirm placental invasion. Particular note should be made of evidence of invasion into the bladder, bowel, or lateral parametria. Intraoperative or preoperative ultrasonography can be utilized to help map the position of the placenta prior to initiating the uterine incision. Hysterotomy should be planned to avoid placental disruption, often necessitating a fundal or posterior hysterotomy. If there is no clear invasion of the placenta into the uterus, manual extraction may be attempted. If there is clear invasion of the placenta into the uterine wall, the placenta should be left in situ and the hysterotomy expeditiously closed so hysterectomy can be initiated or expedient abdominal closure for a planned interval hysterectomy can be completed. Towel clamps for traction and a large, running suture can be used to facilitate closure. Once the hysterotomy is completed and relative hemostasis is obtained, the abdominal contents should be packed with the aid of a self-retaining retractor.

Hysterectomy is initiated with division of the round ligaments or incising the lateral pelvic peritoneum lateral and parallel to the infundibulopelvic ligaments to gain access to the retroperitoneum (Figure 6.2). Once access to the retroperitoneum has been established, the paravesical and pararectal spaces may be opened, the ureters and major pelvic vessels should be identified, and the presence of the ureteral stents and intravascular balloon catheters may be confirmed. Preoperative placement of retrograde ureteral stents may facilitate identification of the ureters at the time of hysterectomy.[7,32] Ureteral stent placement may be particularly helpful in women with placenta accreta and lateral invasion of the placenta into the parametrium. In a series of peripartum hysterectomies performed for placenta accreta, ureteral stent placement reduced early morbidity and decreased the rate of ureteric injury from 7% to 0%.[7]

The utero-ovarian ligaments are transected and the ovaries preserved and packed away. The vesico-uterine peritoneum is then opened and the bladder dissected away from the uterus. In cases of placenta accreta, the placenta bulges into the back wall of the bladder. Vasculature along the lower uterine segment is usually prominent and every attempt should be made to avoid disrupting the placenta. Attention is then turned back to the retroperitoneum. The lateral wall of the uterus is often thin and attenuated making clamp placement difficult. Ligation of the uterine vasculature within the retroperitoneum may help decrease blood loss during the hysterectomy. If possible, the uterine artery and vein can be ligated just distal to origin of the uterine artery from the anterior division of the hypogastric artery. Ligation of the vessels in the retroperitoneum can also facilitate dissection of the ureters in cases where there is placental involvement of the parametrium. Newer generation vessel sealing devices are often helpful in achieving excellent hemostasis on large, vascular pedicles. Dissection should be continued along the cardinal ligament until the uterus is freed to below the level of the placental attachment. The uterus with the placenta can then be amputated and the remainder of the hysterectomy completed in a routine fashion. The choice between total and subtotal hysterectomy should be individualized. While subtotal hysterectomy may be faster, removal of the entire lower uterine segment and cervix may be required to control bleeding.[2,9] A number of studies found no difference in morbidity and operative times between the two procedures.[2,24,33] If the placenta invades the bladder, partial cystectomy may be required. The integrity of the ureters and bladder should be confirmed before closing the abdomen in all patients.

Intraoperative Considerations for Patients with Expected Placenta Accreta

Blood Component Therapy

Major blood loss during a peripartum hysterectomy for a known placenta accreta should be expected and planned for. Immediate availability of blood component therapy is mandatory. For patients in whom hemorrhage is anticipated (placenta accreta), 20 units of cross-matched PRBCs, 20 units of FFP, and 12 units of platelets should be available in the operating suite. As blood loss is often underestimated, early initiation of transfusion is prudent. Vital sign derangements such as tachycardia or hypotension (especially in young women) or the presence of heavy bleeding in the operative field suggest major hemorrhage. Early and ongoing communication with the anesthesia team and operating room personnel is essential.

Traditional guidelines for transfusion protocols recommend an FFP to PRBC ratio of 1:3 with six units of platelets once 10 units of PRBCs have been administered. While data from patients with obstetric hemorrhage are lacking, studies of trauma patients suggest that higher FFP to PRBC ratios may prevent coagulopathy and improve survival.[34,35] A multicenter review of over 450 trauma patients reported that 30-day survival was improved in patients who received a high FFP:PRBC ratio ($\geq$1:2) in comparison to patients that were transfused with a low FFP:PRBC ratio (<1:2).[34] It is recommended to begin transfusion of all major obstetric hemorrhage cases with a 1:1 ratio of FFP to PRBCs.

Cell Salvage Technology

Autologous blood cell salvage devices (cell salvage) may be used at the time of peripartum hysterectomy to minimize transfusion requirements.[36] Cell salvage with reinfusion is less costly than homologous blood, reduces infectious risks and provides immediate access to blood when there is a delay in the availability of homologous blood. While cell salvage could theoretically contain fetal debris, adverse reactions from auto transfusions have not been substantiated. However, there is the possibility of isoimmunization against antigens like Duffy, Kell, or Kidd.[37] There are several obstetric studies that demonstrate safety of the technology.[38-41] The use of cell salvage has been advocated by the ACOG for use in pregnant women when massive transfusion is anticipated.[42]

Procoagulant Technology

A number of topical hemostatic agents are currently available in the United States to promote hemostasis.[43] While data are predominately based on small studies, these agents are being employed in a number of surgical disciplines and may be used as an adjunct to control bleeding in women who undergo peripartum hysterectomy. Topical absorbable agents include microfibrillar collagens, gelatins, and oxidized cellulose. The gelatin-based products including Gelfoam (Pharmacia, Kalamazoo, MI) and Surgifoam (Ethicon, Somerville, NJ) are porcine gelatin sponges that can be placed on surgical surfaces. These products cause platelet adherence and clot formation and can be soaked in thrombin prior to placement. Oxidized regenerated cellulose (Surgicel, Ethicon, Somerville, NJ) also consists of a matrix to facilitate clotting. Flowable matrix agents such as FloSeal (bovine gelatin and thrombin) (Baxter BioSurgery, Fremont, CA) and SurgiFlo (porcine gelatin) (Ethicon, Somerville, NJ) contain granules of collagen or gelatin that expand upon contact with blood to promote tamponade. Fibrin sealants provide fibrin and thrombin to promote the clotting cascade. Tisseel (Baxter BioSurgery, Fremont, CA) is composed of human fibrinogen and thrombin from pooled plasma with bovine aprotinin. Evicel (Ethicon, Somerville, NJ) is a similar product that contains fibrinogen and human thrombin. Synthetic, recombinant activated factor VII (rFVIIa) promotes coagulation in the presence of tissue factor at sites of active bleeding. While rFVIIa is approved in the United States for bleeding associated with hemophilia A and in patients with inhibitors of coagulation, the drug is being increasingly used for other causes of hemorrhage. Although publication bias is likely, rFVIIa has been used in a number of cases of postpartum hemorrhage with reported success rates of >70%.[44] The cost of rFVIIa is often tens of thousands of dollars per patient and should only be used in cases of intractable hemorrhage.

Intravascular Balloon Catheters and Pelvic Artery Embolization

The role of routine placement of internal iliac catheters by interventional radiology or vascular surgery for either temporary balloon occlusion or arterial embolization is controversial. The rationale for temporary balloon inflation during peripartum hysterectomy is to reduce bleeding, improve visualization, and allow for a more controlled operative procedure. There have been multiple reports demonstrating the potential benefit of temporary balloon occlusion.[45-48] In a recent prospective observational study of women with morbidly adherent placenta, the use of balloon catheters decreased both blood loss and transfusion requirements. The benefit attributable to the use of the balloon catheters was most evident in cases of placenta percreta.[46] Despite these encouraging data, there are some reports showing no difference in outcomes.[49,50] There are also several reports cautioning against the routine use of temporary balloon inflation at the time of peripartum hysterectomy due to the risk of significant complications including arterial thrombosis with acute limb ischemia, bladder and rectal wall necrosis, sciatic nerve ischemia, hematoma formation, pseudoaneurysms, and cauda equina syndrome.[51–53] A proper random-ized controlled trial with the power to study the potential benefit of temporary balloon occlusion and its associated complications is unlikely due to the rare occurrence of accreta. Currently, ACOG has argued that "current evidence is insufficient to make a firm recommendation on the use of balloon catheter occlusion or embolization to reduce blood loss and improve surgical outcome, but individual situations may warrant their use."[27] Therefore, the decision to proceed with balloon occlusion or embolization should be at the discretion of the surgical team and should be reserved for cases where significant intra-operative hemorrhage is encountered.

Pelvic Pressure Packing

For patients with hemorrhage refractory to more conservative measures, the abdomen can be closed with laparotomy sponges left in situ. A number of modifications of packing have been reported including an umbrella pack in which a bag is filled with gauze sponges, packed in the pelvis, and placed under traction with a weight brought through the vagina.[54] If the abdomen is packed, patients are usually left intubated and taken back to the operating room for washout and removal of the packing in 1–3 days after aggres-sive correction of the coagulopathy. Aggressive correction of coagulopathy usually provides improved hemostasis when the patient is re-explored to remove packing and wash out the abdomen.

Aortic Compression and Clamping

Aortic compression during instances of massive pelvic hemorrhage can decrease blood flow to the pelvis, allowing the surgical team to gain control of the operative field and giving the anesthesia team criti-cal time for resuscitation with fluid and blood products. If aortic compression or clamping is utilized, the potential for distal thrombosis and ischemia should be considered and vascular surgery should be consulted.[55]

Surgical Management of Limited (Focal) Accreta

Data describing the management of partial or a focal placenta accreta are limited. Placenta accreta occurs when the placenta is abnormally adherent to the myometrium as a result of partial or complete deficiency of the decidua basalis and ineffective Nitabuch's layer. The severity of abnormal placentation depends on the number of placental cotyledons that have adhered to the uterine wall and how deeply they are embedded. It has been argued that there is little clinical difference among women with total, partial, or focal accreta since outcomes are similar. Despite these limitations, some women with focal abnormal placentation may be candidates for uterine-preserving therapies.

The sonographic finding of suspected focal interruptions of the myometrial border (suspected partial accreta) represent a clinical and diagnostic challenge. The optimal management of partial or a focal placenta accreta is uncertain and many institutions utilize different strategies. Due to difficulties in accurately determining the extent and degree of invasion of the placenta, most of these cases should still be performed with a multidisciplinary approach and follow institutional protocols.

Most focal accretas are diagnosed at the time of delivery when the contracting myometrium fails to shear the placenta spontaneously from the uterus. Manual attempts to develop a cleavage plane between the placenta's adherent bed and the uterus to extract the placental mass can result in substantial hemor-rhage. Once the placenta is removed in fragments, it causes a defect in the uterine wall and massive bleeding. In 2004, Kayem et al. studied the impact of maternal outcome of manual placental extraction versus management with the placenta in situ and found a significant reduction in the blood transfusions, disseminated intravascular coagulation (DIC), and hysterectomies when the placenta was left in situ.[56]

In general, removal of the placenta manually should be avoided. It may be reasonable if the diagnosis of an accreta is unknown to the provider or it is a known focal accreta with minimal invasion and other alternatives have been considered. Retained placental fragments not identified at the time of the delivery may cause delayed postpartum bleeding. Although hysterectomy traditionally has been the definitive treatment for placenta accreta, clinicians may consider other medical or surgical management for patients with a focal accreta and who are clinically stable and wish to preserve fertility (see Chapter 7).

Women with a focal accreta who desire future fertility may be candidates for uterine sparring treatment in highly selected scenarios. In these patients, the placenta is separated and medical interventions undertaken to obtain hemostasis and avoid hysterectomy. Hemodynamic instability at any point during attempted conservative management should prompt hysterectomy.

Uterotonics are used with conservative management to maintain uterine contraction and decrease bleeding. After the placenta separates from the myometrium, there may be profuse bleeding from the placental bed. Application of intrauterine pressure with tamponade through either pressure packing or a balloon device may be useful. Using a balloon catheter to control tamponade of the vessels to achieve hemostasis by reducing uterine blood flow is a conservative procedure that is safe, quick, and effective.[57] The successful use of balloon devices has been reported with the Sengstaken–Blakemore esophageal catheter and the Bakri balloon. Advantages of these devices include ease of insertion, painless removal, and rapid identification of treatment failures.[58] This method for the management of postpartum hemorrhage should be performed in patients with stable vital signs in whom persistent bleeding is not excessive.

Opponents of conservative management suggest that it increases the risk of unpredictable sudden massive hemorrhage and/or infection that may result in emergent surgery. Medical techniques are useful when there has been a full separation of the placenta but there is a focal area with an attached placenta that is not deep. Sharp curettage of the area in question also may aid in removal of the placental mass. Surgical repair of myometrial defects may be attempted with oversew of the placental bed to gain hemostasis. Other methods described are the lower uterine segment being everted to remove placental fragments and compression sutures placed as needed for hemostasis. The myometrial defect is then closed in the same way as a hysterotomy.

A variety of reports have described more conservative management of focal placenta accreta. Conservative surgical strategies for women with focal placenta accreta typically rely on local resection with reconstruction of the uterus. In 2004, Palacios et al. proposed an en bloc resection of the entire placental bed. This technique is performed if 50% or less of the anterior uterine circumference of invaded myometrium is involved.[59] The affected area was excised and the myometrial defect covered with myometrial pulley sutures, similar to horizontal mattress sutures, also known as U stiches. The defect was then covered with absorbable vicryl mesh coated with a nonadhesive cellulose layer. Uterine conservation was completed in 50 of the 68 women (74%). Of these, 10 became pregnant and were delivered at 36 weeks by scheduled cesarean delivery 26% still required hysterectomy. No data were reported about the safety of pregnancy or long-term mesh complications.[59]

In 2006, Chandraharan et al. reported the Triple-P procedure on four patients with good outcomes. Once the fetus was delivered, uterine blood supply was reduced with the inflation of prepositioned occlusion balloons in the anterior division of the internal iliac artery. At the time of surgery, a transverse hysterotomy was executed two fingerbreadths above the placental edge and once delivery is achieved the balloons are inflated or uterine artery ligation was performed. The placenta was removed with en bloc myometrial excision and uterine repair with a 2-cm margin of myometrium that was preserved to allow hysterotomy closure of the "myometrial defect."[60] This technique involves the preoperative localization of the placental borders and preoperative placement of intra-arterial balloon catheters. The adherent placental excision and myometrial reconstruction are controversial due to possible complications and morbidity.

While reports have described the successful management of focal accreta with resection and uterine reconstruction, data remain limited. While medical management and conservative resection can be considered, hysterectomy should still be considered the standard approach to management in these women and any evidence of hemodynamic instability should prompt immediate hysterectomy.

Surgical Management of Unexpected Placenta Accreta

The surgical management of unexpected placenta accreta represents a major challenge. As described above, preoperative preparation and the availability of a multidisciplinary team are cornerstones of the successful management of the morbidly adherent placenta. By definition, when an unexpected placenta accreta is encountered, these resources are generally not immediately available.

An unexpected placenta accreta is often grossly obvious at the time of laparotomy. Placental tissue normally distorts the lower uterine segment and may protrude anteriorly, posteriorly, or laterally through the uterus. In contrast, occasionally bleeding may be encountered after extraction of a placenta in which gross uterine invasion was not identified. Regardless, when a morbidly adherent placenta is suspected at the time of operation, the provider should perform a rapid assessment of the uterus, placenta, and surrounding pelvic structures.

The expected course of management depends on two factors, the amount of bleeding and stability of the mother, and the availability of resources. In women who are not actively bleeding and who are hemodynamically stable, hysterotomy should be delayed until resources can be mobilized. In this scenario, blood products should be readied and surgical support called for. Anesthesia support should be mobilized for placement of additional vascular access. As most women are likely to have had regional anesthesia, induction of general anesthesia may be required. Once resources are readied, hysterotomy can be performed away from the placenta. Throughout, the maternal condition should be the first priority.[4]

An alternative approach is required in those women who are not actively bleeding and who are receiving care in centers that cannot mobilize adequate resources for the management of placenta accreta in a timely manner. In this scenario, consideration should be given to closure of the abdomen and maternal transport to a tertiary care center with expertise in the management of placenta accreta.

If a patient is actively bleeding or hemodynamically unstable, efforts should be directed to immediately stabilize the patient. Resuscitation with crystalloid and blood products should begin immediately and the operating room staff mobilized to provide help. Pressure can be applied to actively bleeding surfaces although care should be taken to avoid greater disruption of the placenta. Blood flow to the pelvis can be reduced through aortic compression, either with direct pressure or through cross-clamping. If there is active bleeding, exposure should be maximized with conversion of the Pfannenstiel skin incision to either a Maylard or Cherney or through vertical extension of the incision. The difficulty in managing an unexpected placenta accreta highlights the importance of preoperative diagnosis and treatment planning.[4]

Surgical Management of Second-Trimester Accreta

Placenta accreta is an extremely serious condition that often leads to severe complications at the time of termination of pregnancy (TOP). There are few data that address the management of placenta accreta in the setting of second-trimester spontaneous or induced abortion; most data are derived from case reports or small case series that describe management strategies used and subsequent outcomes. Most guidelines and management recommendations are extrapolated from the management of third-trimester accreta and postpartum hemorrhage management protocols.

In 1995, Rashbaum et al. reported that the likelihood of encountering placenta accreta during a second-trimester termination was 0.04%, which is similar to term pregnancy.[61] Most published cases were diagnosed or occurred at the time of dilation and evacuation (D&E) or hysterectomy.[61–65] To date, there are limited reports of placenta accreta encountered during medical abortion.

Like third-trimester deliveries, abnormal placentation during the second trimester may be unexpected and result in heavy bleeding at the time of termination, or it may be suspected based on abnormal imaging. Preprocedure planning is tantamount when suspicious imaging is encountered in women contemplating second-trimester termination. The patient should be counseled regarding treatment options and a multidisciplinary team assembled to care for the patient and prepare for potential complications. An important consideration for most women with second-trimester accreta is the preservation of future fertility. If further pregnancies are desired, the patient needs to be counseled extensively about the risk of recurrent placental abnormalities in future pregnancies.

There are two management options for women with suspected second-trimester placenta accreta who desire termination: immediate gravid hysterectomy or D&E (Figure 6.3). D&E allows for preservation of fertility and is often successful even in the presence of apparent abnormal placentation on imaging. Hysterectomy should be performed if bleeding is encountered at the time of D&E and conservative measures fail. Alternatively, gravid hysterectomy with the fetus in situ can be performed. This approach may limit blood loss but results in permanent loss of fertility. The primary treatment approach is based on a number of factors as described below and should be individualized.

Women who have completed childbearing can be counseled about both treatment options including a planned hysterectomy. If accreta is suspected and fertility is not desired, the safest way to proceed may be with a planned gravid hysterectomy. The patient should be counseled thoroughly regarding the risks and benefits of hysterectomy, including the risks of emergent obstetric hysterectomy versus planned hysterectomy and the likelihood of success of more conservative measures based on the limited data available. If emergent hysterectomy is required, the procedure is associated with greater blood loss and greater transfusion requirements.[66] For patients with complex comorbid medical conditions who are

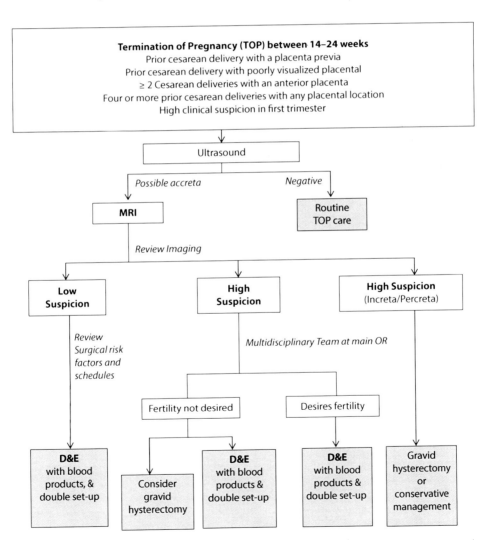

FIGURE 6.3 Flowchart for management of women with suspected second-trimester placenta accreta.

undergoing termination for medical indications, it may be prudent to perform a planned hysterectomy over D&E to avoid the possibility of a hemorrhage in a patient that may not sustain a massive blood loss.[65]

Many institutions will administer intracardic potassium chloride prior to planned termination with gravid hysterectomy or D&E. This may allow compliance with state regulations and also allow time for procedural planning. If D&E is chosen as the method of termination, the procedure should be performed in a setting in which hysterectomy can be expeditiously undertaken if bleeding is encountered and the D&E deemed unsuccessful. Preoperative placement of uterine artery embolization (UAE) catheters can be considered to help control hemorrhage if it is encountered. The use of UAE in the second trimester remains controversial.[63] It is unclear whether UAE should be performed after the procedure if hemorrhage occurs or prior to D&E to decrease the likelihood of hemorrhage and emergent hysterectomy.[64]

If an unexpected placenta accreta is encountered intraoperatively that cannot be resolved quickly with placental extraction and fertility is desired, placement of a Bakri balloon or Foley catheter balloon to provide compression can be attempted.[63,64] Additional hemorrhage prevention strategies used in second-trimester cases include use of uterotonics and uterine massage.[63] If none of the steps for postabortal hemorrhage is successful and UAE is unavailable or unsuccessful, hysterectomy should be performed. The operating room should be prepared with instrumentation and staffing for hysterectomy in all patients with suspicious imaging findings who undergo D&E.

The use of mifepristone and misoprostol for retained adherent placenta after term delivery has recently been described with the successful expulsion of retained placenta several weeks after delivery with no complications.[67] Mifepristone and misoprostol have fewer potential complications than methotrexate, and while their use has not been described as a primary approach to second-trimester abortion with known accreta, it may be an alternative to conservative management with methotrexate, especially given the uncertain benefits and considerable risks of methotrexate. Further study is needed before a conclusion can be made. Currently, there is no evidence that supports the use of methotrexate either prior to D&E or after D&E if the placenta is retained or in lieu of D&E. Mifepristone and misoprostol have been used successfully in some cases of retained adherent placenta at term and may be useful in the management of second-trimester abortion with accreta.

Regardless of the decision to proceed with gravid hysterectomy or D&E, it is paramount that second-trimester abortion cases in which accreta is highly suspected take place in hospital settings in which a multidisciplinary team can be assembled. Ideally, the team is assembled preoperatively and includes participants from family planning, gynecology, oncology, anesthesia, IR, blood bank, and nursing staff to maximize patient safety and outcome.

Perioperative Outcomes and Care

Peripartum hysterectomy is associated with significant morbidity and mortality. Case series suggest that the perioperative mortality rate associated with peripartum hysterectomy ranges from 1% to 7.[3,68] The procedure is also associated with a high rate of adverse outcomes. When compared to morbidities associated with nonobstetric hysterectomy, the perioperative, cardiovascular, pulmonary, gastrointestinal, renal, and infectious morbidities resulting from peripartum hysterectomy are all higher.[3] These complications result in an ICU admission rate of 25%–50%.[69]

One of the most common complications of placenta accreta is hemorrhage that often requires massive transfusion. In a study of 1,798 women with placenta accreta, 48.6% of patients required a transfusion.[3] Similarly, in a retrospective analysis of maternal morbidity in cases of placenta accreta managed by a multidisciplinary team, Eller et al. reported that 82% of patients received one or more units of PRBCs and 43% received four or more units of PRBCs despite being cared for at a Center of Excellence.[5] Various definitions of massive blood transfusion have been described. Some of these definitions include replacement of one entire blood volume within 24 hours, transfusion of greater than 10 units of PRBCs in 24 hours, transfusion of greater than 20 units of PRBCs in 24 hours, transfusion of greater than four units of PRBCs in 1 hour when ongoing need is foreseeable, and replacement of 50% of total blood volume within 3 hours.[18]

An analysis of peripartum hysterectomy from the United Kingdom reported a median transfusion requirement of 10 units of PRBCs and four units of FFP.[2] A retrospective review of 77 patients who underwent hysterectomy for pathologically confirmed placenta accreta reported that the median blood loss was 3 L, with a median of five units of PRBCs transfused. The authors of this study noted that 42% of the cases had an estimated blood loss (EBL) of ≥5L, and 13% of the cases had an EBL of 10 L.[8]

Unfortunately, there are few reliable parameters to predict massive hemorrhage associated with accreta. Therefore, timely intraoperative assessment of the patient's hemodynamic status and laboratory parameters should lead to the expedient use of blood products when massive bleeding is encountered. As reviewed by Belfort, recent data in nonobstetric patients suggests that, in the setting of large hemorrhage, the administration of FFP and platelets in a 1:1 ratio with PRBCs can result in a more rapid correction of coagulopathy, decreased need for PRBC transfusion, and reduced mortality.[55] The California Maternal Quality Care Collaborative published transfusion guidelines for the use in massive obstetric hemorrhage recommending a RBC to plasma to single donor platelets ratio of 6:4:1. They also recommend cryoprecipitate if the patient's fibrinogen level falls below 100 mg/dL.[18] Targets of resuscitation in massive blood loss include a mean arterial pressure (MAP) of around 60 mmHg, hemoglobin of 7–9 g/dL, international normalized ratio (INR) <1.5, activated partial thromboplastin time (aPTT) <42 seconds, platelets >50,000, pH of 7.35–7.45, and a core temperature of >35.0°C.

Complications arising from massive transfusion can be immediate or delayed. Perhaps the most profound complication is inadequate resuscitation leading to hypoperfusion resulting in lactic acidosis, systemic inflammatory response syndrome, DIC, and eventual multiorgan failure. Massive transfusion and volume replacement also increases the risk of circulatory overload and interstitial edema that may lead to compartment syndrome and dilutional coagulopathy. There are also complications that are related directly to the transfusion of large volumes of stored blood. These include citrate toxicity, hyperkalemia, hypothermia, hypomagnesemia, and acidosis. Late or delayed complications from massive transfusion include respiratory failure, transfusion-related acute lung injury, systemic inflammatory response syndrome (SIRS), sepsis, and thrombotic complications.[70]

The most common intraoperative complication from the surgical management of placenta accreta is bladder injury. The rate of bladder injury has been reported to range from 15% to 43%[3,5] and may be even higher in women with placenta percreta. The reason for such high rates of injury are due to a combination of factors including, but not limited to, placental invasion into the bladder, unintentional injury due to poor visualization during surgery, and intentional injury to facilitate adequate bladder dissection and repair if necessary. The estimated prevalence of ureteral injury during hysterectomy for placenta accreta has been reported as high as 10%–15%.[68] However, in a large population-based study, the incidence of ureteral injury in cases of peripartum hysterectomy for accreta was only 1%.[3] Delayed urologic complications that may be seen after hysterectomy for accreta include urinary fistula, small capacity bladder, and ureteral stenosis.

Other intraoperative and perioperative complications include intestinal injury, vascular injury, wound complications, reoperation, venous thromboembolism, pelvic abscess, wound infections, and prolonged hospital and ICU stays. Currently, there are no guidelines clearly defining which patients require admission to the ICU after hysterectomy for accreta and hospital protocols and practices vary. Clear indications include prolonged need of mechanical ventilation, persistent hypotension requiring vasoactive medications, coagulopathy and severe anemia, and any evidence of renal, cardiac, and other end organ dysfunction. If none of these indications exists, transfer to the ICU should remain at the discretion of the surgical and anesthesia teams, and is dependent on institutional practices.

Conclusions

As our understanding of the optimal management of placenta accreta evolves, more data will help refine currently available surgical algorithms that are based on expert opinion. Given the complexity of management, suspicion of abnormal placentation should lead to prompt evaluation. Those women with morbidly adherent placenta should be managed at a center with a multidisciplinary team and experience in treating placenta accreta. Thoughtful preoperative planning, the availability of adequate resources, and involvement of a multidisciplinary team can help reduce the morbidity of women with placenta accreta.

REFERENCES

1. Whiteman MK, Kuklina E, Hillis SD et al. Incidence and determinants of peripartum hysterectomy. *Obstet Gynecol.* 2006;108:1486–1492.

2. Knight M, UKOSS Peripartum hysterectomy in the UK: Management and outcomes of the associated haemorrhage. *BJOG.* 2007;114:1380–1387.

3. Wright JD, Devine P, Shah M et al. Morbidity and mortality of peripartum hysterectomy. *Obstet Gynecol.* 2010;115:1187–1193.

4. Silver RM, Fox KA, Barton JR et al. Center of excellence for placenta accreta. *Am J Obstet Gynecol.* 2015;212:561–568.

5. Eller AG, Bennett MA, Sharshiner M et al. Maternal morbidity in cases of placenta accreta managed by a multidisciplinary care team compared with standard obstetric care. *Obstet Gynecol.* 2011;117:331–337.

6. Shellhaas CS, Gilbert S, Landon MB et al. The frequency and complication rates of hysterectomy accompanying cesarean delivery. *Obstet Gynecol.* 2009;114:224–229.

7. Eller AG, Porter TF, Soisson P, Silver RM. Optimal management strategies for placenta accreta. *BJOG.* 2009;116:648–654.

8. Wright JD, Pri-Paz S, Herzog TJ et al. Predictors of massive blood loss in women with placenta accreta. *Am J Obstet Gynecol.* 2011;205:38.e1–6.

9. Langdana F, Geary M, Haw W, Keane D. Peripartum hysterectomy in the 1990s: Any new lessons? *J Obstet Gynaecol.* 2001;21:121–123.

10. Finberg HJ, Williams JW. Placenta accreta: Prospective sonographic diagnosis in patients with placenta previa and prior cesarean section. *J Ultrasound Med.* 1992;11:333–343.

11. Berkley EM, Abuhamad AZ. Prenatal diagnosis of placenta accreta: Is sonography all we need? *J Ultrasound Med.* 2013;32:1345–1350.

12. Pilloni E, Alemanno MG, Gaglioti P et al. Accuracy of ultrasound in antenatal diagnosis of placental attachment disorders. *Ultrasound Obstet Gynecol.* 2016;47:302–307.

13. Bowman ZS, Eller AG, Kennedy AM et al. Interobserver variability of sonography for prediction of placenta accreta. *J Ultrasound Med.* 2014;33:2153–2158.

14. Levine D, Hulka CA, Ludmir J, Li W, Edelman RR. Placenta accreta: Evaluation with color Doppler US, power Doppler US, and MR imaging. *Radiology.* 1997;205:773–776.

15. Lax A, Prince MR, Mennitt KW, Schwebach JR, Budorick NE. The value of specific MRI features in the evaluation of suspected placental invasion. *Magn Reson Imaging.* 2007;25:87–93.

16. Tanaka YO. MRI of the female pelvis: Useful information for daily practice. *Nihon Lgaku Hoshasen Gakkai Zasshi Nippon Acta Radiologica.* 2002;62:471–478.

17. Maldjian C, Adam R, Pelosi M, Pelosi M, 3rd. MRI appearance of cervical incompetence in a pregnant patient. *Magn Reson Imaging* 1999;17:1399–1402.

18. Stotler B, Padmanabhan A, Devine P, Wright J, Spitalnik SL, Schwartz J. Transfusion requirements in obstetric patients with placenta accreta. *Transfusion.* 2011;51:2627–2633.

19. Estella NM, Berry DL, Baker BW, Wali AT, Belfort MA. Normovolemic hemodilution before cesarean hysterectomy for placenta percreta. *Obstet Gynecol.* 1997;90:669–670.

20. Kruskall MS, Leonard S, Klapholz H. Autologous blood donation during pregnancy: Analysis of safety and blood use. *Obstet Gynecol.* 1987;70:938–941.

21. Silver RM, Landon MB, Rouse DJ et al. Maternal morbidity associated with multiple repeat cesarean deliveries. *Obstet Gynecol.* 2006;107:1226–1232.

22. O'Brien JM, Barton JR, Donaldson ES. The management of placenta percreta: Conservative and operative strategies. *Am J Obstet Gynecol.* 1996;175:1632–1638.

23. Kwee A, Bots ML, Visser GH, Bruinse HW. Emergency peripartum hysterectomy: A prospective study in The Netherlands. *Eur J Obstet Gynecol Reprod Biol.* 2006;124:187–192.

24. Yucel O, Ozdemir I, Yucel N, Somunkiran A. Emergency peripartum hysterectomy: A 9-year review. *Arch Gynecol Obstet.* 2006;274:84–87.

25. Martin JA, Hamilton BE, Sutton PD, Ventura SJ, Menacker F, Munson ML. Births: Final data for 2003. *National Vital Statistics Rep.* 2005;54:1–116.

26. Stafford IA, Dashe JS, Shivvers SA, Alexander JM, McIntire DD, Leveno KJ. Ultrasonographic cervical length and risk of hemorrhage in pregnancies with placenta previa. *Obstet Gynecol.* 2010;116:595–600.

27. Committee on Obstetric Practice. Committee opinion no. 529: Placenta accreta. *Obstet Gynecol.* 2012;120:207–211.
28. Warshak CR, Ramos GA, Eskander R et al. Effect of predelivery diagnosis in 99 consecutive cases of placenta accreta. *Obstet Gynecol.* 2010;115:65–69.
29. Robinson BK, Grobman WA. Effectiveness of timing strategies for delivery of individuals with placenta previa and accreta. *Obstet Gynecol.* 2010;116:835–842.
30. Gyamfi-Bannerman C, Thom EA, Blackwell SC et al. Antenatal betamethasone for women at risk for late preterm delivery. *N Engl J Med.* 2016;374:1311–1320.
31. Wright JD, Herzog TJ, Shah M et al. Regionalization of care for obstetric hemorrhage and its effect on maternal mortality. *Obstet Gynecol.* 2010;115:1194–1200.
32. Shellhaas CS, Gilbert S, Landon MB et al. The frequency and complication rates of hysterectomy accompanying cesarean delivery. *Obstet Gynecol.* 2009;114:224–229.
33. Kastner ES, Figueroa R, Garry D, Maulik D. Emergency peripartum hysterectomy: Experience at a community teaching hospital. *Obstet Gynecol.* 2002;99:971–975.
34. Holcomb JB, Wade CE, Michalek JE et al. Increased plasma and platelet to red blood cell ratios improves outcome in 466 massively transfused civilian trauma patients. *Ann Surg.* 2008;248:447–458.
35. Borgman MA, Spinella PC, Perkins JG et al. The ratio of blood products transfused affects mortality in patients receiving massive transfusions at a combat support hospital. *J Trauma.* 2007;63:805–813.
36. Catling S, Joels L. Cell salvage in obstetrics: The time has come. *BJOG.* 2005;112:131–132.
37. Fong J, Gurewitsch ED, Kump L, Klein R. Clearance of fetal products and subsequent immunoreactivity of blood salvaged at cesarean delivery. *Obstet Gynecol* 1999;93:968–972.
38. Sullivan I, Faulds J, Ralph C. Contamination of salvaged maternal blood by amniotic fluid and fetal red cells during elective Caesarean section. *Br J Anaesth.* 2008;101:225–229.
39. Waters JH, Biscotti C, Potter PS, Phillipson E. Amniotic fluid removal during cell salvage in the cesarean section patient. *Anesthesiology.* 2000;92:1531–1536.
40. Allam J, Cox M, Yentis SM. Cell salvage in obstetrics. *Int J Obstet Anesth.* 2008;17:37–45.
41. Catling S. Blood conservation techniques in obstetrics: A UK perspective. *Int J Obst Anesth.* 2007;16:241–249.
42. American College of Obstetricians and Gynecologists. ACOG Practice bulletin: Clinical management guidelines for obstetrician-gynecologists number 76, October 2006: Postpartum hemorrhage. *Obstet Gynecol.* 2006;108:1039–1047.
43. Pursifull NF, Morey AF. Tissue glues and nonsuturing techniques. *Curr Opin Urol.* 2007;17:396–401.
44. Alfirevic Z, Elbourne D, Pavord S et al. Use of recombinant activated factor VII in primary postpartum hemorrhage: The Northern European registry 2000-2004. *Obstet Gynecol.* 2007;110:1270–1278.
45. Carnevale FC, Kondo MM, de Oliveira Sousa W Jr. et al. Perioperative temporary occlusion of the internal iliac arteries as prophylaxis in cesarean section at risk of hemorrhage in placenta accreta. *Cardiovasc Intervent Radiol.* 2011;34:758–764.
46. Cali G, Forlani F, Giambanco L et al. Prophylactic use of intravascular balloon catheters in women with placenta accreta, increta and percreta. *Eur J Obstet Gynecol Reprod Biol.* 2014;179:36–41.
47. Dubois J, Garel L, Grignon A, Lemay M, Leduc L. Placenta percreta: Balloon occlusion and embolization of the internal iliac arteries to reduce intraoperative blood losses. *Am J Obstet Gynecol.* 1997;176:723–726.
48. Shih JC, Liu KL, Shyu MK. Temporary balloon occlusion of the common iliac artery: New approach to bleeding control during cesarean hysterectomy for placenta percreta. *Am J Obstet Gynecol.* 2005;193:1756–1758.
49. Bodner LJ, Nosher JL, Gribbin C, Siegel RL, Beale S, Scorza W. Balloon-assisted occlusion of the internal iliac arteries in patients with placenta accreta/percreta. *Cardiovasc Intervent Radiol.* 2006;29:354–361.
50. Levine AB, Kuhlman K, Bonn J. Placenta accreta: Comparison of cases managed with and without pelvic artery balloon catheters. *J Matern Fetal Med.* 1999;8:173–176.
51. Mok M, Heidemann B, Dundas K, Gillespie I, Clark V. Interventional radiology in women with suspected placenta accreta undergoing caesarean section. *Int J Obstet Anesth.* 2008;17:255–261.
52. Teare J, Evans E, Belli A, Wendler R. Sciatic nerve ischaemia after iliac artery occlusion balloon catheter placement for placenta percreta. *Int J Obstet Anesth.* 2014;23:178–181.

53. Greenberg JI, Suliman A, Iranpour P, Angle N. Prophylactic balloon occlusion of the internal iliac arteries to treat abnormal placentation: A cautionary case. *Am J Obstet Gynecol.* 2007;197:470. e1–4.

54. Howard RJ, Straughn JM Jr., Huh WK, Rouse DJ. Pelvic umbrella pack for refractory obstetric hemorrhage secondary to posterior uterine rupture. *Obstet Gynecol.* 2002;100:1061–1063.

55. Publications Committee SfM-FM, Belfort MA. Placenta accreta. *Am J Obstet Gynecol.* 2010;203:430–439.

56. Kayem G, Davy C, Goffinet F, Thomas C, Clement D, Cabrol D. Conservative versus extirpative management in cases of placenta accreta. *Obstet Gynecol.* 2004;104:531–536.

57. Ferrazzani S, Guariglia L, Triunfo S, Caforio L, Caruso A. Conservative management of placenta previa-accreta by prophylactic uterine arteries ligation and uterine tamponade. *Fetal Diagn Ther.* 2009;25:400–403.

58. Doumouchtsis SK, Papageorghiou AT, Arulkumaran S. Systematic review of conservative management of postpartum hemorrhage: What to do when medical treatment fails. *Obstet Gynecol Surv.* 2007;62:540–547.

59. Palacios Jaraquemada JM, Pesaresi M, Nassif JC, Hermosid S. Anterior placenta percreta: Surgical approach, hemostasis and uterine repair. *Acta Obstet Gynecol Scand.* 2004;83:738–744.

60. Chandraharan E, Rao S, Belli AM, Arulkumaran S. The triple-P procedure as a conservative surgical alternative to peripartum hysterectomy for placenta percreta. *Int J Gynaecol Obstet.* 2012;117:191–194.

61. Rashbaum WK, Gates EJ, Jones J, Goldman B, Morris A, Lyman WD. Placenta accreta encountered during dilation and evacuation in the second trimester. *Obstet Gynecol.* 1995;85:701–703.

62. Yang JI, Kim HY, Kim HS, Ryu HS. Diagnosis in the first trimester of placenta accreta with previous Cesarean section. *Ultrasound Obstet Gynecol.* 2009;34:116–118.

63. Steinauer JE, Diedrich JT, Wilson MW, Darney PD, Vargas JE, Drey EA. Uterine artery embolization in postabortion hemorrhage. *Obstet Gynecol.* 2008;111:881–889.

64. Borgatta L, Chen AY, Reid SK, Stubblefield PG, Christensen DD, Rashbaum WK. Pelvic embolization for treatment of hemorrhage related to spontaneous and induced abortion. *Am J Obstet Gynecol.* 2001;185:530–536.

65. Tocce K, Thomas VW, Teal S. Scheduled hysterectomy for second-trimester abortion in a patient with placenta accreta. *Obstet Gynecol.* 2009;113:568–570.

66. Doumouchtsis SK, Arulkumaran S. The morbidly adherent placenta: An overview of management options. *Acta Obstet Gynecol Scand.* 2010;89:1126–1133.

67. Morgan M, Atalla R. Mifepristone and misoprostol for the management of placenta accreta—A new alternative approach. *BJOG.* 2009;116:1002–1003.

68. Silver RM, Barbour KD. Placenta accreta spectrum: Accreta, increta, and percreta. *Obstet Gynecol Clin North Am.* 2015;42:381–402.

69. Bretelle F, Courbiere B, Mazouni C et al. Management of placenta accreta: Morbidity and outcome. *Eur J Obstet Gynecol Reprod Biol.* 2007;133:34–39.

70. Patil V, Shetmahajan M. Massive transfusion and massive transfusion protocol. *Indian J Anaesth.* 2014;58:590–595.

7

Conservative Management of Placenta Accreta

Loïc Sentilhes, Gilles Kayem, and Robert M. Silver

CONTENTS

Introduction

Conservative management of placenta accreta is defined as all procedures or strategies aiming to avoid a peripartum hysterectomy and its related morbidity and consequences. The main goals are to (1) decrease severe maternal morbidity related to the placental disease, especially the amount of blood loss (in turn, this decreases the risk of massive transfusion and coagulopathy as well as operative injury, mainly bladder and ureteral injury, and its potential consequences such as vesicouterine fistula) and (2) attempt to preserve the option of future pregnancies, knowing that fertility is often inextricably linked with societal status and self-esteem. Four main types of conservative management have been described: (1) extirpative treatment,[1] (2) expectant management or leaving the placenta in situ,[2] (3) one-step conservative surgery,[3] and (4) the Triple-P procedure.[4]

The Extirpative Approach

The concept of this approach is simple: the aim is to avoid leaving retained placental tissue in the uterine cavity. Retained placenta is a common cause of postpartum hemorrhage (PPH), and complete removal decreases the risk of bleeding.[5–12] The procedure consists of manually removing the placenta to obtain an "empty" uterus. Unfortunately, in cases of morbidly adherent placenta (MAP), this procedure often results in massive hemorrhage. Kayem et al. performed a retrospective study comparing two consecutive periods. In the first one, the extirpative approach was routinely applied for MAP, whereas in the second one, the placenta was left in situ. Mean number of red blood cells (RBC) transfused ($3,230 \pm 2,170$ mL vs. $1,560 \pm 1,646$ mL; $p < 0.01$), disseminated intravascular coagulation

(5 [38.5%] vs. 1 [5.0%]; $p = 0.02$), and hysterectomy rates (11 [84.6%] vs. 3 [15%]; $p < 0.001$)were reduced using the placenta in situ approach.[1] Moreover, when a cesarean-hysterectomy for suspicion of MAP has been planned, Eller et al. have shown that the early maternal morbidity was increased when a placental removal was attempted compared with the placenta left undisturbed in situ (67% vs. 36%; $p = 0.04$).[13] Consequently, several authorities recommend that manual placental removal should be avoided in cases of planned cesarean-hysterectomy.[14–16] The downside of this approach is the potential for unnecessary hysterectomy if the patient does not really have MAP. In conclusion, extirpative approach with a forcible manual removal of the placenta should be abandoned unless the probability of MAP is low.[17] Unfortunately, manual removal of the placenta usually happens in most cases with undiagnosed placenta accreta. In our opinion, women with strongly suspected MAP should never have an attempted manual removal of the placenta. For women with risk factors for MAP or even a mild suspicion of MAP, caregivers should stop attempts to manually remove the placenta in cases of unusual and unexplained difficulties before the occurrence of massive hemorrhage.

Leaving Placenta In Situ or Expectant Management

Short- and Mid-Term Maternal Outcome

This approach consists of leaving the placenta in situ and waiting for complete resorption. It was first described mainly in France[2] and initially was termed "conservative treatment of placenta accreta." As other conservative approaches have been since described, it is more accurate to use the term "leaving the placenta in situ" or "expectant management."[18]

The goals of this approach are to avoid the morbidity associated with hysterectomy, preserve fertility, and still avoid hemorrhage. Cesarean-hysterectomy is considered the gold standard treatment for MAP[11–17] but is associated with high rates of severe maternal morbidity (40%–50%).[17] Cesarean-hysterectomy with placenta percreta is even more morbid, with reported mortality rates up to 7%.[19] By leaving the MAP in situ after the delivery of the child, one can expect a significant decrease of blood flow within the uterus and even the parametrium. This also will occur within the placenta, and the placenta will progressively and spontaneously detach from the uterus and even adjacent organs by necrosis. It is analogous to cutting the foot of an ivy plant that is incrusted into a stone wall and waiting for it to die before removing it in order to avoid weakening the stone wall. This approach is particularly attractive for severe MAP with adjacent organ invasion in order to avoid operative complications and injuries.

On the other hand, expectant management has significant risks. These include intrauterine infection, placental abscess, and even sepsis, as well as unpredictable massive hemorrhage. Moreover, it requires long-term monitoring until complete resorption of the placenta occurs.

In practice, the exact position of the placenta is determined by a preoperative ultrasound. Before initiating cesarean delivery, all materials required for an immediate conversion to hysterectomy are readily available (Figure 7.1a). Laparotomy is made by a midline cutaneous incision, often enlarged above the umbilicus (Figure 7.1c). The uterine approach uses a midline or "classical" incision at a distance from the placental bed (Figure 7.1d). After the delivery of the child, and only in cases wherein MAP is unlikely, the obstetrician carefully attempts to remove the placenta by controlled cord traction (see later in this section). If the placenta does not easily separate from the uterus, it confirms the diagnosis of MAP. In this case, the cord is cut at the site of insertion (Figure 7.1e), and the uterine cavity is closed (Figure 7.1f). Postoperative antibiotic therapy (amoxicillin and clavulanic acid) is usually administered prophylactically for 5 days to minimize the risk of infection, although efficacy is uncertain. Adjunctive procedures (embolization [Figure 7.1g] or vessel ligation, temporal internal iliac occlusion balloon, methotrexate, hysteroscopic resection of retained tissues) may be used to attempt to decrease morbidity or to hasten placental resorption. As with antibiotic treatment, none of these interventions has been proven to improve outcomes.

In France, the first conservative treatment took place in 1993; the number of procedures increased steadily, particularly during the 2000s.[4] First, only very limited data about maternal outcome after

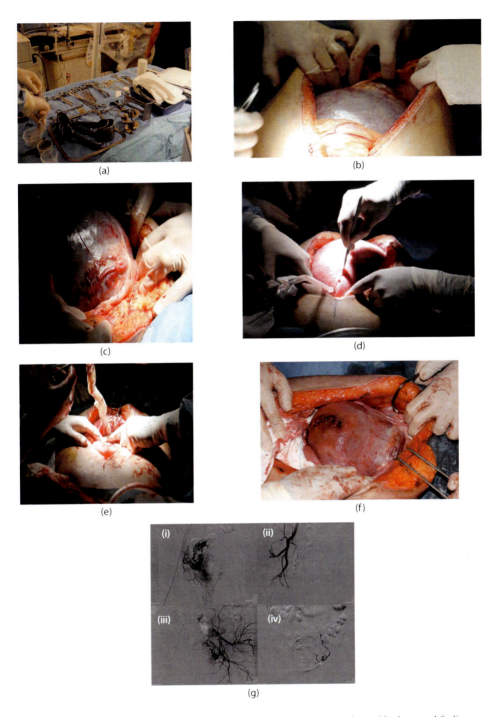

FIGURE 7.1 (a) A 28-year-old patient with a history of two previous cesarean sections with ultrasound findings conclusive to a morbidly adherent placenta (MAP) opted for conservative management, but all material required for an immediate conversion to hysterectomy is ready on an adjacent table. (b) View of the abdominal cavity after a midline cutaneous incision, enlarged above the umbilicus. (c) Perioperative view that confirms the diagnosis of MAP. (d) Midline incision at a distance from the placental bed. (e) Umbilical cord is cut at the site of insertion after the delivery of the child with no attempt at placental removal due to the perioperative confirmation of the diagnosis of MAP. (f) Perioperative view of MAP left in situ after the closing of the vertical fundal uterine incision. (g) Angiograms before and after a prophylactic pelvic arterial embolization for MAP of the right (i, ii) and left (iii, iv) sides. Note the significant decrease of the vascularization at the end of the procedure.

conservative management were available. Moreover, they were from small case reports and case series from individual tertiary-care institutions.[1,20,21]

In 2007, Timmermans et al. reviewed available case series of placenta accreta managed by leaving the placenta in situ.[22] They found 48 case reports describing the outcome of 60 women as well as two French case series reporting including 31 women yielding available data on 91 cases. Of the 26 women managed conservatively while leaving the placenta in situ without the use of additional therapies, 22 (85%) had a favorable outcome. Expectant management failed in 4 (15%) of the patients who required hysterectomy due to severe hemorrhage or infection.[22]

In order to increase statistical power and satisfactory external validity, a French multicenter retrospective study was conducted to determine the maternal outcome after conservative treatment.[2] Of the 45 university hospitals in France, 40 (88.9%) agreed to participate in the study and 25 used conservative treatment for placenta accreta at least once.

Placenta accreta was diagnosed according to the following clinical and histologic criteria: (1) It was partially or totally impossible to manually remove the placenta with no discernable cleavage plane between all or part of the placenta and uterus. (2) Prenatal diagnosis of placenta accreta on sonogram (Figure 7.2a), confirmed by the failure of gentle attempts to remove it during the third stage of labor or at cesarean delivery. (3) Evidence of placental invasion at the time of surgery (Figures 7.1b and 7.2b). (4) Histologic confirmation of accreta on hysterectomy specimen. Women treated with an extirpative approach or a planned cesarean-hysterectomy were excluded from this study. Conservative management in case of placenta accreta was defined by the decision of the obstetrician to leave the placenta partially or totally in situ, with no attempt to remove it forcibly (Figures 7.1f and 7.2c). When placenta accreta was not suspected before delivery, it was diagnosed when it was impossible to detach the placenta by gentle manipulation, and conservative treatment was defined as leaving part or all of it in the uterus.

The study included 167 cases of placenta accreta with 59% of placentas left partially in situ and 41% left totally in situ. Outcomes are summarized in Table 7.1.[2] Success rates were similar to prior reports[4,20] with uterine preservation (no hysterectomy) in 78.4% of cases and severe maternal morbidity in only 6% (10/167) (defined as any of the following: sepsis, septic shock, peritonitis, uterine necrosis, postpartum uterine rupture, fistula, injury to adjacent organs, acute pulmonary edema, acute renal failure, deep vein thrombophlebitis or pulmonary embolism, or maternal death).[2] One maternal death related to multiorgan failure occurred in a patient with aplasia, nephrotoxicity with acute renal failure, followed by peritonitis with septic shock, after injection of methotrexate in the umbilical cord. Other rare morbidities included vesicovaginal fistula and arteriovenus fistula formation. These complications also have been reported by others.[23–25]

The placenta spontaneously and completely resorbed in 75% of cases after a median of 13.5 weeks (minimum: 4 weeks, maximum: 60 weeks) (Figure 7.2d through 7.2m). Hysteroscopic resection and/or curettage were performed to remove any remaining placenta in 25% with a median of 20 weeks (minimum: 2 weeks, maximum: 45 weeks).[2] Strengths of this retrospective study included a large number of cases studied and participating centers, which increased the study's external validity and made it possible to extrapolate the results to other university teaching hospitals that may have limited experience in conservative treatment of placenta accreta but where blood banks, pelvic arterial embolizations, obstetric subspecialties, obstetric anesthesia, interventional radiology, urology, and gynecological oncology are readily available. Limitations include its retrospective design and the absence of histologic confirmation of MAP in cases without hysterectomy. Accordingly, some of these cases may not truly have been MAP, resulting in an underestimation of maternal morbidity associated with conservative management. Indeed, only about half of women had a placenta previa and a prenatal suspicion of MAP.[17] This problem of MAP definition concerns all studies related to placenta accreta/increta/percreta when no hysterectomy specimen is available and makes assessment of conservative management of MAP difficult. In this study, we used stringent and uniformly applied criteria to define MAP (see earlier in this section) in order to minimize this limitation. Also, we confirmed MAP on histopathological examination in all primary hysterectomies (18/18) and all except one delayed hysterectomy (17/18).

TABLE 7.1

Maternal Morbidity after Conservative Treatment for Placenta Accreta

Characteristics	Placenta Accreta, Including Percreta (n = 167)
Placenta left in situ	167 (100)
Partially	99 (59.3)
Entirely	68 (40.7)
Primary postpartum hemorrhage (PPH)	86 (51.5)
No additional uterine devascularization procedure	58 (34.7)
Additional uterine devascularization procedure	109 (65.3)
Pelvic arterial embolization[a]	62 (37.1)
Vessel ligation[a]	45 (26.9)
Stepwise uterine devascularization	15 (9.0)
Hypogastric artery ligation	23 (13.8)
Stepwise uterine devascularization and hypogastric artery ligation	7 (4.2)
Uterine compression suture[a]	16 (9.6)
Balloon catheter occlusion	0
Methotrexate administration	21 (12.6)
Primary hysterectomy	18 (10.8)
Cause of primary hysterectomy	
Primary PPH	18/18 (100)
Postpartum prophylactic antibiotic therapy > 5 days	54 (32.3)
Transfusion patients	70 (41.9)
Units of packed red blood cells transfused > 5	25 (15.0)
Transfer to intensive care unit	43 (25.7)
Infection	47 (28.1)
Septic shock	1 (0.6)
Sepsis	7 (4.2)
Vesicouterine fistula	1 (0.6)
Uterine necrosis	2 (1.2)
Deep vein thrombophlebitis or pulmonary embolism	4 (2.4)
Secondary PPH	18 (10.8)
Delayed hysterectomy	18 (10.8)
Median interval from delivery to delayed hysterectomy	22 (9–45)
Cause of delayed hysterectomy	
Secondary PPH	8/18 (44.4)
Sepsis	2/18 (11.1)
Secondary PPH and sepsis	3/18 (16.7)
Vesicouterine fistula	1/18 (5.6)
Uterine necrosis and sepsis[b]	2/18 (11.1)
Arteriovenous malformation	1/18 (5.6)
Maternal request	1/18 (5.6)
Death	1 (0.6)
Success of conservative treatment	131 (78.4)
Severe maternal morbidity	10 (6.0)

Source: Sentilhes L et al., *Obstet Gynecol,* 115, 526–534, 2010.

Notes: Data presented as mean ± standard deviation, or as median with interquartile range in parentheses, or as number of patients with percentages in parentheses. Some patients had more than one type of morbidity. Success of conservative treatment was defined as uterine preservation. A primary hysterectomy took place within the first 24 hours, whereas a delayed hysterectomy took place more than 24 hours after delivery.

[a] The total number of additional uterine devascularization procedures exceeds the number of patients because some patients had more than one such procedure.

[b] These two patients had bilateral supra-selective embolization of the uterine arteries due to primary PPH on the day of delivery.

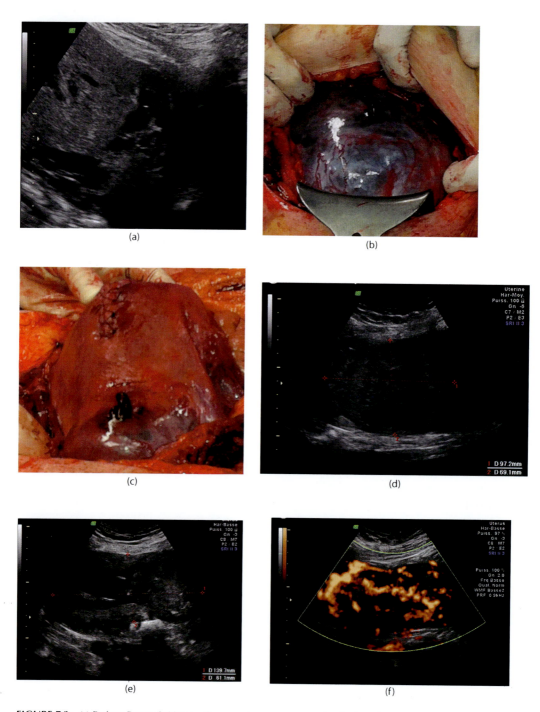

FIGURE 7.2   (a) Patient: Parous 2, history of one previous cesarean section for breech presentation, prenatal ultrasonography with conclusive findings of MAP (numerous placenta lacunae, thinning or disruption of hyperechoic serosa bladder interface, irregular retroplacental sonolucent zone); opted for an attempt of leaving in situ approach. (b) Perioperative view that confirms the diagnosis of MAP. (c) Perioperative view of MAP left in situ after the closing of the vertical fundal uterine incision. (d) Day 15 after delivery: Presence of a voluminous homogenous placental mass in the uterine cavity. (e) Day 30 after delivery: Onset of placental resorption with in homogenous placental mass that remains voluminous. (f) Day 30 after delivery: Persistence of rich placental vascularization on color Doppler energy.

(Continued)

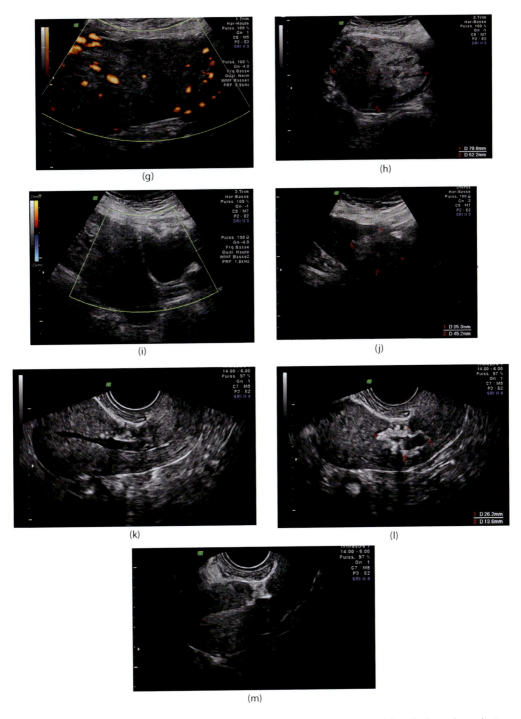

FIGURE 7.2 (*Continued*) (g) Day 45 after delivery: Persistence of a large retained placental tissue in the uterine cavity (more than 10 cm of great diameter) with a significant vascularization decrease on color Doppler energy. (h) Day 120 after delivery: Significant decrease of the size of retained placental tissue. (i) Day 120 after delivery: Reappearance of a normal hyperechoic serosa bladder interface. (j) Day 150 after delivery: Reappearance of a normal continuous white line at the top of the fundus with persistent retained placenta in the previous lower uterine segment with a great diameter of 45 mm. (k) Day 180 after delivery: Uterine cavity empty; menstruation resumed. (l) Day 180 after delivery: Uterine cavity empty with a persistent hyperechoic scar in the myometrium of the previous lower uterine segment. (m) Day 210 after delivery: Persistent hyperechoic scar in the myometrium of the previous lower uterine segment and into the previous uterine scar related to the first cesarean section.

Data are even more scarce regarding conservative management of placenta percreta. Pather et al. reported three cases of placenta percreta with conservative management and also performed a review of available data. They found 57 cases of suspected placenta percreta that were managed conservatively with the placenta left in situ. Hysterectomy was avoided in 60% of cases and 42% experienced major morbidity (including sepsis, coagulopathy, hemorrhage, pulmonary embolism, fistula, and arteriovenous malformation).[26] In a similar review, Clausen et al. retrieved 36 cases of placenta percreta managed by leaving the placenta in situ.[23] Delayed hysterectomy was required in 58% of cases. In a French national study that reported the largest series of consecutive cases of placenta percreta with attempt to leave the placenta in situ ($n = 18$), prenatal diagnosis by ultrasonography or magnetic resonance imaging (MRI) was performed in 14 cases and during labor (at the time of the cesarean) in four cases.[2] Conservative treatment was successful for 10 of 18 cases (55.6%) of placenta percreta, and severe maternal morbidity occurred in 3 of the 18 (16.7%). Of the 8 cases of placenta percreta with bladder involvement, conservative treatment was successful in 6 cases (75%), and severe maternal morbidity occurred in 2 (25%).[2] Although morbidity was considerable, it was favorable in comparison with similar cases with planned cesarean-hysterectomy.[19]

These results show that leaving placenta in situ is a reasonable option for women who are properly counseled and motivated, in particular, if they desire future pregnancies. It also is critical that they agree to close follow-up monitoring in centers with adequate equipment and resources.[2,11–17] However, many questions remain unanswered:

- Should a routine gentle attempted removal (by only doing a gentle traction on the umbilical cord) of the placenta be made in cases of suspected prenatal placenta accreta?

The main drawback of this strategy is that attempted removal of the placenta can cause severe bleeding with the risk of maternal hemorrhagic complications and hysterectomy. The main advantage is to potentially avoid leaving an in situ placenta, if there is not really MAP, as well as to remove the "non-accreta" portion of the placenta when the placenta adheres partially to the myometrium. This can reduce the volume of placenta left in the uterus, potentially reducing the risk of bleeding and infection. It is important to emphasize imprecision in the antenatal diagnosis of MAP using Doppler ultrasound and/or MRI. These two imaging modalities are good but imperfect for the diagnosis of MAP.[26] The consequences of a false-negative result are obvious, i.e., increased maternal morbidity.[27–29] Similarly, caregivers should be aware that false-positive results, which may occur in up to 28% of cases,[13] also increase maternal morbidity. These false-positive results may lead caregivers to perform unnecessary radical or conservative surgical procedures that may also result in possible complications. It makes sense to consider the context. Thus, our current practice is to attempt to gently remove the placenta by cord traction only in cases when the diagnosis of placenta accreta is uncertain. An example would be a nulliparous woman with a history of curettage for whom ultrasound revealed intraplacental lacunae in a low-lying anterior placenta and no visible evidence of placenta accreta during the cesarean.[17]

- Should methotrexate adjuvant treatment be administered?

Some authors have proposed the use of methotrexate to hasten placental resolution.[30] Its efficacy for this indication has never been demonstrated and only case reports and small case series with no control groups have been reported.[22] Accordingly, the Royal College of Obstetricians and Gynaecologists (RCOG) does not recommend its routine use.[16] The low rate of placental cell division in the third trimester compared to early pregnancy raises the question of whether methotrexate has any effect on placental resorption. In addition, methotrexate rarely causes serious harm such as neutropenia or medullary aplasia, even with a single dose in a young patient.[31] These complications can have a dramatic impact in a patient with an intra-uterine placenta with a 30% risk of infectious complications.[2] Finally, the only case, to our knowledge, of maternal death after conservative treatment was secondary to a cascade of complications (bone marrow suppression, sepsis, renal failure) attributed to an intra-umbilical cord administration of methotrexate.[2] For these reasons, we do not advocate the use of methotrexate in cases of conservative treatment.

- Should preventive uterine devascularization be carried out in the absence of bleeding?

There are few data available to answer this question. Preventive devascularization can be achieved by techniques used to treat PPH (embolization, bilateral uterine artery ligation, stepwise uterine devascularization, bilateral ligation of hypogastric arteries), although these uterine-sparing procedures may be less effective in cases of placenta accreta.[32,33] Angstmann et al. demonstrated that preventive embolization before performing cesarean-hysterectomy may reduce the risk of blood loss with accreta.[34] Thus, it is possible that prophylactic devascularization could reduce the risk of secondary hemorrhage in the setting of conservative treatment (Figure 7.1g).[35] It could also theoretically accelerate placental resolution. In fact, in a retrospective comparative study, the median delay for complete placental resorption was significantly shorter when women underwent an embolization (median = 17 weeks; $q_1$011.5; $q_3$023; range: 1–38 weeks) compared to women who do not undergo embolization (median = 32 weeks; $q_1$018; $q_3$048.8; range: 12–111 weeks) (p = 0.036). Unfortunately, the reason for embolization was not clearly reported by the authors.[36] In contrast, devascularization may cause harm.[2,33] In the French multicenter series of 167 placenta accreta treated conservatively, the only two cases of uterine necrosis occurred in 2 of 62 patients who underwent arterial embolization.[2] Other adverse effects of uterine artery embolization also have been reported.[37] The risk:benefit ratio of routine devascularization procedures in conservative management of placenta accreta remains to be determined.

- How should patients with conservative management be monitored?

Unfortunately, there are no data regarding this important issue. In our practice, we observe the patient in the hospital for 8 days and administer prophylactic antibiotics for 5 days. This window is the time of highest risk for bleeding and infection. Prior to discharge, the woman and her partner should be advised about the need for close, long-term monitoring. There is still a risk for bleeding and infection and the size and vascularization of the retained placenta often does not significantly change for several weeks (Figures 7.2d through 7.2g). The following symptoms require emergency medical attention: hyperthermia, severe pelvic pain, foul-smelling vaginal discharge, and bleeding. The patient also should be advised about the possibility of abnormal and persistent vaginal discharge. There should be a multidisciplinary team available with the skills to manage complications 24 hours a day, 7 days a week. Patients are seen for outpatient clinic visits weekly for the first 2 months. If the patient is asymptomatic, monthly visits are then conducted until complete resorption of the placenta. The visits include a clinical examination (bleeding, temperature, pelvic pain), pelvic ultrasound (size of retained tissue), and laboratory screen for infection (hemoglobin and leukocytes, C-reactive protein, vaginal sample for bacteriological analysis).[2] Of course, the efficacy of these measures is uncertain.

We do not use magnetic resonance (MRI) imaging and beta-human chorionic gonadotropin (β-HCG) level for monitoring. Nevertheless, Soyer et al. used MRI to follow 23 women with placenta left in situ for MAP.[36] The median delay for complete placental resorption was 21.1 weeks (range, 1–111 weeks). They found a significant correlation between the degree of vascularity on early phase of dynamic MRI and delay of complete placental resorption (r = 0.69; p < 0.001). They speculated that MRI may help predict delay for complete placental resorption.[36] It is not clear whether decreasing levels of β-HCG correlate with the rate of involution of placental tissue. Khan et al. and Torrenga et al. reported several cases of placenta left in situ followed by monitoring serum β-HCG levels.[38,39] Serum β-HCG levels decreased to minimal levels in 5 months in the Khan study and in 5–10 weeks in the Torrenga study. In both studies, β-HCG levels did not correlate with the volume of remaining tissue,[38,39] raising questions about its usefulness for the monitoring of these patients.

- Should routine hysteroscopic resection of retained placental tissue be performed?

Again, data regarding this issue are scarce. As mentioned above, in a French retrospective study, either hysteroscopic resection or curettage or both were used to remove retained placenta in 29 (25.0%) cases, at a median of 20 weeks (range: 2–45 weeks) after delivery.[2] These results highlight the fact that this procedure is performed frequently. Nevertheless, no information regarding the reason for performing this procedure (due to pain, bleeding, and/or infection, to hasten placental resorption, on maternal request, or systematically) was available. In a small cohort series of 23 women with placenta left in situ for placenta accreta, 12 had undergone hysteroscopy under ultrasound guidance due to pain and/or bleeding with retained tissues.[40] The use of bipolar energy was limited as much as possible to minimize risk of uterine perforation. The median size of the retained placenta was 54 mm (13–110). No complications occurred due to hysteroscopic resection. Complete removal (11/12) was achieved after one, two, and three hysteroscopic procedures in five (41.7%), two (16.7%), and four (33.3%) cases, respectively. One delayed hysterectomy was performed after "failure" of the hysteroscopic procedure.[40] It seems that hysteroscopic resection may shorten recovery time without harmful effects in symptomatic women. The role of prophylactic hysteroscopy or the timing of it in asymptomatic women is unknown.

- Should systematic delayed interval hysterectomy be planned?

A possible advantage of leaving the placenta in situ is to plan a delayed interval hysterectomy after partial involution of the placenta and decreased uterine vascularity. This may decrease hemorrhagic morbidity and risk of injury to adjacent organs. This strategy seems most attractive in women with placenta percreta, who are at highest risk for blood loss and urinary tract injury. Excellent outcomes have been reported using this approach in percreta cases.[41] On the other hand, this approach requires two surgeries instead of one, and both may be quite morbid. Also, there is a risk of hemorrhage or infection prompting the need for emergency hysterectomy during the planned interval. Finally, the optimal timing of planned delayed hysterectomy is uncertain.[1] It may only be possible to truly ascertain whether delayed interval hysterectomy is effective through appropriate clinical trials.

Long-Term Maternal Outcome and Subsequent Fertility and Obstetrical Outcome

Few data are available regarding subsequent pregnancies in women with conservative management of MAP using the placenta in situ approach, but successful pregnancies have been reported.[21,42] However, these reports are biased toward successful outcomes. Therefore, an attempt was made to contact all women included in the French national retrospective study who did not undergo a hysterectomy, to estimate fertility and pregnancy outcomes after successful expectant management.[43] Follow-up data were available for 96 (73.3%) of the 131 women included in the study. There were eight women who had severe intrauterine synechiae and were amenorrheic. Of the 27 women who wanted more children, 3 women were attempting to become pregnant (mean duration: 11.7 months, range: 7–14 months), and 24 (88.9%) women had had 34 pregnancies (21 third-trimester deliveries, 1 ectopic pregnancy, 2 elective abortions, and 10 early pregnancy losses) with a mean time to conception of 17.3 months (range: 2–48 months). All 21 deliveries resulted in healthy babies born after 34 weeks of gestation. Placenta accreta recurred in 6 of 21 cases (28.6%) and was associated with placenta previa in four cases. PPH occurred in four (19%) cases, related to placenta accreta in three and to uterine atony in one. These results show that successful expectant management for placenta accreta can be associated with successful subsequent fertility and pregnancy, although there is an increased risk of recurrent MAP.[43]

Cesarean-Hysterectomy or Conservative Treatment?

There is only one small retrospective study comparing maternal outcome following cesarean-hysterectomy ($n = 16$) vs. placenta in situ conservative management ($n = 10$).[44] No differences were observed between groups except for estimated blood loss, which was lower in the conservative treatment group (3625 mL ± 2154 vs. 900 mL ± 754; $p < 0.05$).[44] Of course, this study was too small and prone to bias to truly compare strategies. In fact, it is possible that severe maternal morbidity is increased in cases of conservative treatment because unpredictable infectious complications, uterine necrosis, and secondary hemorrhage associated with conservative treatment can be dramatic. As with delayed interval hysterectomy, the relative merits of planned cesarean-hysterectomy and conservative management will only be elucidated through properly designed clinical trials.

Until such trials are completed, it seems reasonable to counsel women about planned cesarean-hysterectomy and conservative management. A major consideration is whether or not future childbearing is desired. A planned cesarean-hysterectomy may be the best option if the patient has no desire for more children, is older, and/or multiparous. Nevertheless, we believe that conservative management is a reasonable option for patients who are properly counseled and motivated, for example, women who want the option of future pregnancies, who agree to close follow-up monitoring, and who are in centers with adequate equipment and resources.[1–2,11,17,45]

Moreover, leaving the placenta in situ may be the most appropriate choice in the most severe cases of MAP, in particular, in cases of organ adjacent invasion,[46] where radical surgery is often associated with severe maternal morbidity.[19] Others also favor this approach, even in the United States where conservative management is less common than in France. A recent US survey noted that 14.9% of providers would attempt to leave the placenta in situ in a hemodynamically stable patient[47] and 32% had attempted conservative management for placenta accreta.[48]

One-Step Conservative Surgery

One-step conservative surgery is an alternative conservative procedure that has been described by one author.[49–51] It consists of resecting the invaded area of the uterus together with the placenta and reconstructing the uterus. It is done at the time of cesarean delivery as a "one-step procedure."[50] This strategy aims to combine the advantages of the leaving the placenta in situ approach (i.e., preserving fertility) and of cesarean-hysterectomy (no persistent high risk of bleeding or infection after the procedure). The main steps of this uterine-sparing technique achieved through a median or Pfannenstiel incision are (1) vascular disconnection of newly formed vessels and the separation of invaded uterine from invaded vesical tissues, (2) performance of an upper-segmental hysterotomy, (3) resection of all invaded tissue and the entire placenta in one piece, (4) use of surgical procedures for hemostasis, (5) myometrial reconstruction in two planes, and (6) bladder repair if necessary.[51]

Palacios-Jaraquemada et al. described outcomes of this one-step conservative surgery on 68 women presenting with placental invasion of adjacent organs (invasion of the posterior upper bladder section [$n = 46$; group 1] and of the posterior lower vesical section [$n = 22$; group 2]).[49] Uterine preservation was achieved in 95.7% (44/46) and 27.3% (6/22) of cases, respectively. The indications for the 18 hysterectomies were segmental circumferential rupture greater than 50% ($n = 13$), coagulopathy ($n = 2$), infection ($n = 1$), and uncontrolled hemodynamic instability ($n = 2$). The following complications were reported (mostly in group 2): lower ureteral injuries ($n = 2$), vesical fistula ($n = 1$), hematoma in the vaginal cuff ($n = 1$), and uterine infection ($n = 1$). Among the 50 women with uterine preservation, follow-up was available in 42. Menses were recovered between 3 and 16 months. Ten women had another uneventful pregnancy and delivery with no recurrence of MAP.[49] In another publication, Palacios-Jaraquemada et al. reported 45 pregnancies following a one-step procedure for placenta accreta.[50] Of these 45 pregnancies, 44 were uneventful and only one was complicated by a recurrence of placenta accreta.[50]

As we have limited experience with the one-step conservative surgery,[52] we find it difficult to have a clear opinion regarding the technique. It is important to note that the one-step procedure may be less reproducible than conservative treatment because it requires a novel and specific surgical procedure. Successful use of the procedure by other groups and prospective trials will ultimately clarify the merits of the one-step conservative therapy.

The Triple-P Procedure

Chandraharan et al. proposed a novel uterine-sparing procedure for MAP called "the Triple-P procedure."[53,54] The main steps of this strategy are (1) preoperative placental localization using transabdominal ultrasound to identify the superior border of the placenta in order to deliver the fetus by an incision above the upper border of the placenta, (2) pelvic devascularization involving preoperative placement of intra-arterial balloon catheters with inflation after delivery, and (3) no attempt to remove the placenta with en bloc myometrial excision and uterine repair. It seems important to ensure that a 2-cm margin of myometrium is retained in the lower lip of the uterine incision to facilitate closure of the myometrial defect.[53] Bleeding from the separated and adherent part of the placenta is controlled by oversewing the defect. If the posterior wall of the bladder is involved, placental tissue invading the bladder is left in situ to avoid cystotomy.

The authors first described the technique performed successfully on four women.[53] They have since reported a larger series, comparing outcomes after ($n = 19$) and prior to implementation of the Triple-P procedure ($n = 11$). In the past, MAP was treated with an elective cesarean delivery, using an incision into the uterine fundus, leaving the placenta in part or entirely in the uterus unless PPH occurred and peripartum hysterectomy was required (control group).[54] Demographic characteristics were comparable between groups, with percreta rate in 54.5% and 68.4% ($p = 0.35$), respectively. There was no statistical difference for the estimated mean blood loss (2,170 mL vs. 1,700 mL; $p = 0.44$) and the rate of transfusion (45.5% vs. 47.4%; $p = 0.61$). However, the rate of PPH (54.5% vs. 15.8%; $p = 0.035$) and hysterectomy (27.3% vs. 0.0%; $p = 0.045$) were lower in the Triple-P group. One major complication (5%) occurred in a woman treated with Triple-P (right common iliac and external iliac artery thrombosis).[52] This is a known complication of temporal internal iliac occlusion balloon catheters.[55] As with the one-step procedure, these data should be considered preliminary, and further studies are needed to assess relative efficacy. It is noteworthy that the Royal College of Obstetricians and Gynaecologists do not recommend balloons for cesarean-hysterectomy or conservative treatment[15] due to untoward effects, although the issue remains controversial.[56]

Conclusions

Except for extirpative treatment, conservative management for placenta accreta has become an alternative valid option to planned cesarean-hysterectomy in well-selected cases, appropriate counseling, and close surveillance. The best-studied conservative approach is expectant care after leaving placenta in situ. However, even this approach is of uncertain efficacy due to bias in case selection and uncertainty regarding the diagnosis of MAP. Prospective trials are desperately needed to assess the true risks and benefits of conservative management overall as well as for each approach. The French prospective PACCRETA study has been launched in order to answer some of the questions raised in this chapter.[57]

Disclosure of Interests

The authors have no direct or indirect commercial financial incentive associated with publishing this chapter.

Contribution to Authorship

Loïc Sentilhes wrote the first draft of the report. All authors contributed to the writing of the final version and to its revision for important intellectual content, and all have seen and approved the final version.

Funding

The authors declare no source of funding.

REFERENCES

1. Kayem G, Davy C, Goffinet F, Thomas C, Clement D, Cabrol D. Conservative versus extirpative management in cases of placenta accreta. *Obstet Gynecol*. 2004;104:531–536.

2. Sentilhes L, Ambroselli C, Kayem G, et al. Maternal outcome after conservative treatment of placenta accreta. *Obstet Gynecol*. 2010;115:526–534.

3. Palacios-Jaraquemada JM, Pesaresi M, Nassif JC, Hermosid S. Anterior placenta percreta: Surgical approach, hemostasis and uterine repair. *Acta Obstet Gynecol Scand*. 2004;83:738–744.

4. Teixidor Viñas M, Belli AM, Arulkumaran S, Chandraharan E. Prevention of postpartum hemorrhage and hysterectomy in patients with morbidly adherent placenta: A cohort study comparing outcomes before and after introduction of the Triple-P procedure. *Ultrasound Obstet Gynecol*. 2015;46:350–355.

5. Royal College of Obstetricians and Gynaecologists. Postpartum hemorrhage: Prevention and management. April 2011. Available at: http://www.rcog.org.uk/womens-health/clinical-guidance/prevention-and-management-postpartum-haemorrhage-green-top-52. Accessed on November 1, 2013.

6. ACOG Practice Bulletin. Clinical management guidelines for obstetricians and gynecologists: Postpartum hemorrhage. Number 76. *Obstet Gynecol*. 2006;108:1039–1047.

7. Royal Australian and New Zealand College of Obstetricians and Gynaecologists. Management of postpartum hemorrhage. March 2011. Available at: http://www.ranzcog.edu.au/collegestatements-guidelines.html. Accessed on November 1, 2013.

8. Leduc D, Senikas V, Lalonde AB, et al. Active management of the third stage of labour: Prevention and treatment of postpartum hemorrhage. *J Obstet Gynaecol Can*. 2009;31:980–993.

9. World Health Organisation. WHO recommendations for the prevention of postpartum haemorrhage. World Health Organisation, Geneva (Switzerland). 2012. Available at: http://apps.who.int/iris/bitstream/10665/75411/1/9789241548502_eng.pdf. Accessed on May 1, 2016.

10. FIGO Safe Motherhood and Newborn Health (SMNH) Committee. Prevention and treatment of post-partum hemorrhage in low-resource settings. *Int J Gynecol Obstet*. 2012;117:108–118.

11. Sentilhes L, Vayssière C, Deneux-Taraux C, et al. Postpartum hemorrhage: Guidelines for clinical practice from the French College of Gynaecologists and Obstetricians (CNGOF) in collaboration with the French Society of Anesthesiology and Intensive Care (SFAR). *Eur J Obstet Gynecol Biol Reprod*. 2016;198:12–21.

12. Kayem G, Keita H. Management of placenta previa and accrete. *J Gynecol Obstet Biol Reprod*. 2014;43:1142–1160.

13. Eller AG, Porter TF, Soisson P, Silver RM. Optimal management strategies for placenta accreta. *BJOG*. 2009;116:648–654.

14. Publications Committee, Society for Maternal-Fetal Medicine, Belfort MA. Placenta accreta. *Am J Obstet Gynecol*. 2010 Nov;203(5):430–439. DOI: 10.1016/j.ajog.2010.09.013.

15. Committee on Obstetric Practice. Committee opinion No. 529: Placenta accreta. *Obstet Gynecol*. 2012;120:207–211.

16. RCOG. *Placenta Praevia, Placenta Praevia Accreta and Vasapraevia: Diagnosis and Management*. London: RCOG (greentop 27); 2011.

17. Sentilhes L, Goffinet F, Kayem G. Management of placenta accreta. *Acta Obstet Gynecol Scand*. 2013;92:1125–1134.

18. Fox KA, Shamshirsaz AA, Carusi D, et al. Conservative management of morbidly adherent placenta: Expert review. *Am J Obstet Gynecol*. 2015;213:755–760.

19. O'Brien JM, Barton JR, Donaldson ES. The management of placenta percreta: Conservative and operative strategies. *Am J Obstet Gynecol*. 1996;175:1632–1637.

20. Bretelle F, Courbiere B, Mazouni C, et al. Management of placenta accreta: Morbidity and outcome. *Eur J Obstet Gynecol Reprod Biol*. 2007;133:34–39.

21. Alanis M, Hurst BS, Marshburn PB, Matthews ML. Conservative management of placenta increta with selective arterial embolization preserves future fertility and results in a favorable outcome in subsequent pregnancies. *Fertil Steril*. 2006;86:1514.e3–7.

22. Timmermans S, van Hof AC, Duvekot JJ. Conservative management of abnormally invasive placentation. *Obstet Gynecol Surv*. 2007;62:529–539.

23. Barber JT Jr, Tressler TB, Willis GS, et al. Arteriovenous malformation identification after conservative management of placenta percreta with uterine artery embolization and adjunctive therapy. *Am J Obstet Gynecol*. 2011;204:e4–8.

24. Sentilhes L, Descamps P, Goffinet F. Arteriovenous malformation following conservative treatment of placenta percreta with uterine artery embolization but no adjunctive therapy. *Am J Obstet Gynecol.* 2011;205(6):e13.

25. Clausen C1, Lönn L, Langhoff-Roos J. Management of placenta percreta: A review of published cases. *Acta Obstet Gynecol Scand.* 2014;93:138–143.

26. Pather S, Strockyj S, Richards A, Campbell N, de Vries B, Ogle R. Maternal outcome after conservative management of placenta percreta at caesarean section: A report of three cases and a review of the literature. *Aust N Z J Obstet Gynaecol.* 2014;54:84–87.

27. Warshak CR, Ramos GA, Eskander R, et al. Effect of predelivery diagnosis in 99 consecutive cases of placenta accreta. *Obstet Gynecol.* 2010;115:65–69.

28. Tikkanen M, Paavonen J, Loukovaara M, Stefanovic V. Antenatal diagnosis of placenta accreta leads to reduced blood loss. *Acta Obstet Gynecol Scand.* 2011;90:1140–1146.

29. Eller AG, Bennett MA, Sharshiner M, et al. Maternal morbidity in cases of placenta accreta managed by a multidisciplinary care team compared with standard obstetric care. *Obstet Gynecol.* 2011;117:311–317.

30. Mussalli GM, Shah J, Berck DJ, Elimian A, Tejani N, Manning FA. Placenta accreta and methotrexate therapy: Three case reports. *J Perinatol.* 2000;20:331–334.

31. Isaacs JD Jr, McGehee RP, Cowan BD. Life-threatening neutropenia following methotrexate treatment of ectopic pregnancy: A report of two cases. *Obstet Gynecol.* 1996;88:694–696.

32. Sentilhes L, Trichot C, Resch B, et al. Fertility and pregnancy outcomes following uterine devascularization for severe postpartum haemorrhage. *Hum Reprod.* 2008;23:1087–1092.

33. Sentilhes L, Gromez A, Clavier E, Resch B, Verspyck E, Marpeau L. Predictors of failed pelvic arterial embolization for severe postpartum hemorrhage. *Obstet Gynecol.* 2009;113:992–999.

34. Angstmann T, Gard G, Harrington T, Ward E, Thomson A, Giles W. Surgical management of placenta accreta: A cohort series and suggested approach. *Am J Obstet Gynecol.* 2010;202:38.e1–9.

35. Bouvier A, Sentilhes L, Thouveny F, et al. Planned caesarean in the interventional radiology cath lab to enable immediate uterine artery embolization for the conservative treatment of placenta accreta. *Clin Radiol.* 2012;67:1089–1094.

36. Soyer P, Sirol M, Fargeaudou Y, et al. Placental vascularity and resorption delay after conservative management of invasive placenta: MR imaging evaluation. *Eur Radiol.* 2013;23:262–271.

37. Poujade O, Ceccaldi PF, Davitian C, et al. Uterine necrosis following pelvic arterial embolization for post-partum hemorrhage: Review of the literature. *Eur J Obstet Gynecol Reprod Biol.* 2013;170:309–314.

38. Khan M, Sachdeva P, Arora R, Bhasin S. Conservative management of morbidly adherant placenta—A case report and review of literature. *Placenta.* 2013;34:963–966.

39. Torrenga B, Huirne JA, Bolte AC, van Waesberghe JH, de Vries JI. Postpartum monitoring of retained placenta. Two cases of abnormally adherent placenta. *Acta Obstet Gynecol Scand.* 2013;92:472–475.

40. Legendre G, Zoulovits FJ, Kinn J, Sentilhes L, Fernandez H. Conservative management of placenta accreta: Hysteroscopic resection of retained tissues. *J Minim Invasive Gynecol.* 2014;21:910–913.

41. Lee PS, Bakelaar R, Fitpatrick CB, Ellestad SC, Havrilesky LJ, Alvarez Secord A. Medical and surgical treatment of placenta percreta to optimize bladder preservation. *Obstet Gynecol.* 2008;112:421–424.

42. Kayem G, Pannier E, Goffinet F, Grange G, Cabrol D. Fertility after conservative treatment of placenta accreta. *Fertil Steril.* 2002;78:637–638.

43. Sentilhes L, Trichot C, Resch B, et al. Fertility and pregnancy outcomes following uterine devascularization for severe postpartum haemorrhage. *Hum Reprod.* 2008;23:1087–1092.

44. Amsalem H, Kingdom JC, Farine D, et al. Planned caesarean hysterectomy versus "conserving" caesarean section in patients with placenta accreta. *J Obstet Gynaecol Can.* 2011;33:1005–1010.

45. Kayem G, Sentilhes L, Deneux-Tharaux C. Management of placenta accreta. *BJOG.* 2009;116:1536–1537.

46. Sentilhes L, Resch B, Clavier E, Marpeau L. Extirpative or conservative management for placenta percreta? *Am J Obstet Gynecol.* 2006;195:1875–1876.

47. Jolley JA, Nageotte MP, Wing DA, Shrivastava VK. Management of placenta accreta: A survey of maternal-fetal medicine practitioners. *J Matern Fetal Neonatal Med.* 2012;25:756–760.

48. Esakoff TF, Handler SJ, Granados JM, Caughey AB. PAMUS: Placenta accreta management across the United States. *J Matern Fetal Neonatal Med.* 2012;25:761–765.

49. Palacios-Jaraquemada JM, Pesaresi M, Nassif JC, Hermosid S. Anterior placenta percreta: Surgical approach, hemostasis and uterine repair. *Acta Obstet Gynecol Scand.* 2004;83:738–744.

50. Palacios-Jaraquemada JM. Diagnosis and management of placenta accreta. *Best Pract Res Clin Obstet Gynecol*. 2008;22:1133–1148.

51. Palacios-Jaraquemada JM. *Placental Adhesive Disorders*. Berlin/Boston, MA: Walter de Gruyter; 2012.

52. Kayem G, Deis S, Estrade S, Haddad B. Conservative management of a near-term cervico-isthmic pregnancy, followed by a successful subsequent pregnancy: A case report. *Fertil Steril*. 2008;89:1826. e13–15.

53. Chandraharan E, Rao S, Belli AM, Arulkumaran S. The Triple-P procedure as a conservative surgical alternative to peripartum hysterectomy for placenta percreta. *Int J Gynaecol Obstet*. 2012;117:191–194.

54. Teixidor Viñas M, Belli AM, Arulkumaran S, Chandraharan E. Prevention of postpartum hemorrhage and hysterectomy in patients with morbidly adherent placenta: A cohort study comparing outcomes before and after introduction of the Triple-P procedure. *Ultrasound Obstet Gynecol*. 2015;46:350–355.

55. Dilauro MD, Dason S, Athreya S. Prophylactic balloon occlusion of internal iliac arteries in women with placenta accreta: Literature review and analysis. *Clin Radiol*. 2012;67:515–520.

56. Izbizky G, Meller C, Grasso M, et al. Feasibility and safety of prophylactic uterine artery catheterization and embolization in the management of placenta accreta. *J Vasc Interv Radiol*. 2015;26:162–169.

57. Kayem G, Deneux-Tharaux C, Sentilhes L, PACCRETA group. PACCRETA: Clinical situations at high risk of placenta ACCRETA/percreta: Impact of diagnostic methods and management on maternal morbidity. *Acta Obstet Gynecol Scand*. 2013;92:476–482.

8

Role of Interventional Radiology in the Management of Abnormal Placentation

Vineet K. Shrivastava, Gladys A. Ramos, and Michael P. Nageotte

CONTENTS

Perhaps the greatest challenge in modern obstetrical care is the surgical management of abnormal placentation. Over the past 4 decades, there has been a 10-fold increase in the incidence of abnormally adherent placenta compromising pregnancy, which essentially comprises placenta accreta (and its variants, increta and percreta). With the recommended course of action in the management of abnormal placentation from the American College of Obstetrics and Gynecology being cesarean hysterectomy, the critical issue of controlling massive hemorrhage at the time of surgery is faced by all those involved in the care of such patients. Recurrent reports suggest this degree of hemorrhage often exceeds 2 L of blood.[1] Several efforts have been made to mitigate this risk as well as other risks associated with these challenging surgeries. One of the most provocative efforts has been assessing the potential for utilizing interventional radiology (IR) in the surgical care of such cases.

Integrating various IR techniques to reduce the amount of uterine and pelvic blood flow and surgical hemorrhage in such patients to both facilitate surgery and decrease risks of morbidity and mortality has been widely employed. The prevailing theory is that a reduction of uterine perfusion allows for a controlled hysterectomy with decreased hemorrhage resulting in reduced surgical complications and patient morbidity and mortality. In addition, placement of intra-arterial catheters allows for embolization of pelvic vessels if bleeding persists following delivery and hysterectomy. While the use of these techniques theoretically shows promise, there has been inconsistency in reports regarding these techniques, particularly when they are used prophylactically. It is important to understand differences among studies, both with respect to the techniques employed and when they are employed and in what patients. Issues such as prophylactic (preoperative) placement of occlusive balloon catheters (OBCs), balloon catheters (BCs) plus embolization, location of OBCs (hypogastric artery vs. common iliac vs. aorta), embolization alone, timing of deployment of OBC, timing and location of embolization procedure, as well as having suspicion preoperatively of abnormal placentation or discovering this during surgery are some of the issues to be considered in any effort to interpret the studies of such techniques in these patients (Table 8.1). Further, issues such as surgical management, completion of hysterectomy, and experience of the surgical team are critical yet often nonquantifiable variables in these cases. To date, there has not been an adequately powered prospective trial of any radiologic interventions addressing the potential benefits of IR techniques in the management of abnormal placentation.

TABLE 8.1

Summary of Literature of Patients with Interventional Radiologic Procedures for Management of Abnormal Adherent Placentas (Organized by Year)

Author	Total Patients (Number with Balloons)	Balloons/ Embolization	Comparison Group	Benefit	Comment
Salim et al. (2015)[15]	27 (13)	Yes/no	Yes— Randomized	No	• Powered to units of blood transfused • Only randomized trial
Cali et al. (2014)[9]	53 (30)	Yes/no	Yes	Yes	• Benefit observed in percretas • No benefit in accreta/increta
Ballas et al. (2012)[8]	117 (59)	Yes/no	Yes	Yes	• Majority of controls not diagnosed antenatally • Only study to deploy balloons situationally vs. routinely
Angstmann et al. (2010)[14]	26 (8)	Yes/yes	Yes*	Yes—from embolization	• Patients in both groups received balloons, difference between groups was embolization*
Tan et al. (2007)[7]	25 (11)	Yes/yes	Yes	Yes	• Notes benefit in blood loss and need for transfusion • No difference in mean hemoglobin change
Shrivastava (2006)[12]	69 (19)	Yes/no	Yes	No	• No difference noted when emergency cases were excluded from control group
Bodner et al. (2006)[13]	28 (6)	Yes/yes	Yes	No	
Penning et al. (2001)[19]	72 (14)	Yes/no	Yes	No	
Levine et al. (1999)[10]	9 (5)	Yes/no	Yes	No	

* Patient in both groups received balloons; the difference between groups was embolization.

Argument Supporting IR Procedures in the Management of Abnormal Placentation

Massive hemorrhage is a complication of the surgical management of abnormal placentation due in no small part to significant collateral blood flow and neovascularization within the uterus and pelvis resulting from an ongoing pregnancy. Given this risk of profound hemorrhage, several different approaches have been investigated in an effort to limit intraoperative blood loss. Such efforts have focused primarily upon reducing blood flow to the pelvic vessels. The internal iliac (hypogastric) arteries and their branches have been targeted with the assumption that intravascular occlusion results in a decrease in pulse pressure distal to the occlusion and potentially results in a decrease in the risks of massive hemorrhage and blood transfusion (Figure 8.1).

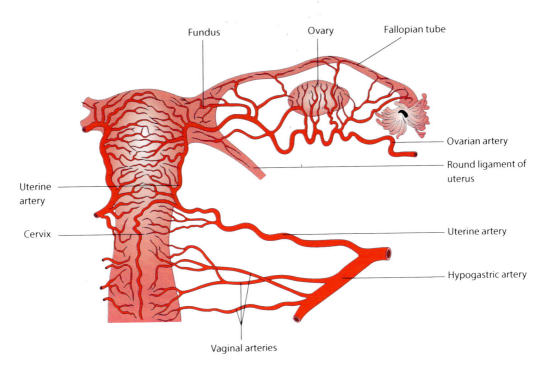

FIGURE 8.1 Uterine blood supply (hypogastric artery).

Arterial embolization to reduce hemorrhage following peripartum hysterectomy to control obstetrical hemorrhage was first reported by Brown et al. in 1979.[2] As a treatment for placenta accreta complicating surgery, uterine artery embolization was first reported by Mitty et al. in 1993.[3] However, reports supporting benefit of such techniques have varied with regard to the actual procedure, the agents used for embolization as well as the timing, and clinical circumstances of the IR procedures. For example, there have been studies utilizing gelfoam or polyvinyl alcohol particles for arterial embolization as primary treatment when hemorrhage persists after hysterectomy versus prospectively during surgery as an adjunct to conservative management (uterine preservation) of placenta accreta.[4] Such comparisons, while interesting, are really not clinically relevant as the surgical procedures are so different. Other reports have aimed to evaluate internal iliac artery (hypogastric) occlusion with BCs placed prior to planned hysterectomy in the setting of placenta accreta. Two retrospective studies reported improved outcomes with the use of OBC of the internal iliac arteries.[5,6] It should be noted that both of these studies lacked a comparison or control group. Carnevale et al. reported their surgical experience with intraoperative temporary deployment of BCs in the internal iliac arteries following cesarean delivery, but prior to hysterectomy in patients with placenta accreta. Twenty-one cases of ultimately confirmed placenta accreta underwent preoperative placement of intravascular catheters by IR. Their technique involved placement of 6-French vascular sheaths in both femoral arteries. BCs (6 or 7 mm) were then placed in the main trunks of the contralateral internal iliac artery. Confirmation of the placement and evidence of vascular occlusion was tested angiographically (Figure 8.2). Balloons were then inflated intraoperatively following delivery of the fetus. These authors reported a significant reduction of blood loss in their patients when compared with a historical control group of accreta patients managed in a similar manner surgically but without OBCs. Of note, they reported two significant vascular complications. The first was a thrombosis of the femoral artery requiring thrombectomy. The second was a thrombus in the external iliac artery. Both complications occurred in women whose surgeries lasted for more than 6 hours. Thon et al. performed a retrospective case series of internal iliac BCs in patients whose delivery required cesarean hysterectomy. Again, there was no control group. They reported improved hemostasis and surgical field visibility in 6 of 11 patients who had internal iliac artery BCs. Importantly, only two of these 11 patients actually had placenta accreta.

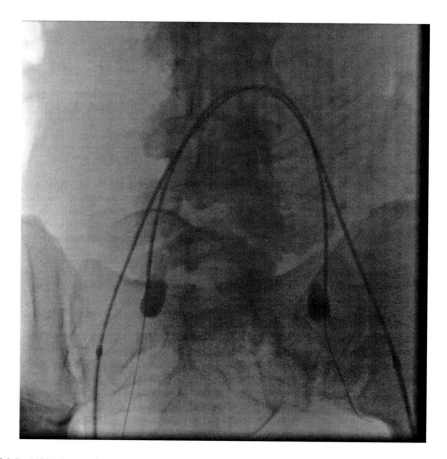

FIGURE 8.2   UCSD image of balloons in bilateral internal iliac arteries.

In a retrospective study using historical controls, Tan et al. reported outcomes in 11 suspected cases of placenta accreta with use of preoperative placement of internal iliac balloons for occlusion.[7] Their technique was similar to Carnevale et al. with inflation of the intravascular balloons immediately following cutting the umbilical cord with delivery of the fetus by cesarean section. Balloons remained inflated until just before skin closure. The treatment group had less mean intraoperative blood loss (2011 mL vs. 3316 mL; $p = 0.04$) with a 52% reduction in the mean volume of blood transfused (1058 mL vs. 2211 mL; $p = 0.005$). However, in addition to the problems associated with using historical controls, not all patients with suspected abnormal placentation had uniform intraoperative management. Specifically, in these 11 cases only four women had a hysterectomy, two had placental removal without hysterectomy, and five had retained placentas without immediate hysterectomy (conservative treatment). These five women also underwent uterine artery embolization with absorbable gelatin sponge following delivery. Two of these five cases developed postpartum hemorrhage with one requiring hysterectomy and one developing disseminated intravascular coagulopathy. The authors concluded that such vascular occlusion was a safe technique associated with lower intraoperative blood loss and transfusion requirement. The risks were as stated but not clearly related to the catheter technique as the management was so different in the two patients with complications.

One of the largest case control publications involving pathologically proven cases of placenta accreta was that of Ballas et al.[8] Cases were divided into those with preoperative internal iliac artery balloon catheter placement (59 patients) and those not so treated (58 patients). They reported a significant reduction in mean blood loss (2165 mL vs. 2837 mL; $p = 0.02$) when internal iliac BCs were placed in anticipation of obstetrical hemorrhage at surgery. In addition, fewer subjects experienced greater than

2500 mL blood loss and fewer patients required massive transfusions (six units or more of packed red blood cells [PRBCs]). No difference was reported in intraoperative complications, length of hospitalization, or intensive care admissions. It is important to note that this study differed from others in that the occlusive balloons were only inflated if it was thought that excessive hemorrhage was being encountered. This commonly was at the time of bladder dissection and/or uterine artery ligation. Another major concern with this report is that essentially all patients who underwent preoperative balloon placement had a prenatal diagnosis of suspected placenta accreta while only 29% had preoperative suspicion of accreta in the historical control group. The strong clinical suspicion preoperatively of abnormal placentation is likely associated with improved patient outcomes as it allows a tailored approach with expectations of potential surgical challenges. In the report by Ballas et al., a subanalysis comparing cases in which balloons were deployed with cases in which they were not revealed a significantly decreased blood loss associated with balloon deployment (1.2 L vs. 2.8 L). However, when the analysis was limited only to patients suspected preoperatively to have abnormal placentation, there were no differences noted in mean blood loss among patients with or without intravascular balloons. Further, there were two significant complications in the study patients, which included a femoral artery thrombus requiring thrombectomy and a catheter site hematoma.

A more recent study that supported the use of OBC was performed by Cali et al.[9] They report 30 subjects who received prophylactic BCs and compared these women with 23 historical controls who had hysterectomy alone and no IR techniques. In this report, all patients were antenatally suspected of having abnormal placentation. Again, there was a reported significant reduction in mean blood loss (846 mL vs. 1156 mL; $p = 0.04$), and a significant reduction in the number of units of blood and blood products transfused. It was also reported that the effect was more pronounced in the more invasive cases of abnormal placentation (i.e., increta and percreta). This study is the first to suggest that the difficulty in demonstrating the value of IR procedures in such patients may be attributed to the severity and heterogeneity of the abnormal placentation.

The lack of consistent reports of improvement with various preoperative interventional radiological concerns has raised the issue of harm. There is concern that inflation of the balloons immediately following delivery in all patients may result in a marked opening of collateral circulation within the pelvis. This could lead to increased blood flow to uterine and cervical vessels resulting in an increased risk of blood loss. Further, as has been reported, such techniques are not free of potential significant vascular morbidity and long-term sequelae.

The Argument Not Supporting IR Procedures in the Management of Abnormal Placentation

Several reports have failed to demonstrate benefit with various preoperative and intraoperative interventional radiological techniques in patients suspected to have abnormal placentation. Levine et al. were the first to report a prospective study of five patients who received prophylactic BCs and had their outcomes compared against historical controls who had an unsuspected diagnosis of placenta accreta.[10,11] In this study, no significant differences in estimated blood loss (5025 vs. 4653 mL), units of packed red cells transfused (5.5 vs. 4), and hospital stay (7 vs. 5 days) were noted among groups. The inherent conflict in this investigation, similar to the Ballas et al. study, was the comparison of antenatally diagnosed vs. intraoperatively diagnosed placenta accreta.

Shrivastava et al. further substantiated these findings in a larger study of 69 subjects, 19 of whom received OBCs.[12] In this study, there were no differences noted in mean estimated blood loss (2700 vs. 3000 mL; $p = 0.79$), number of units transfused (10 vs. 6.5 units; $p = 0.60$), postoperative hospital days (5 vs. 4 days; $p = 0.85$), AND operative time (182 vs. 180 minutes; $p = 0.85$). As with previous studies, the hysterectomy alone group included a mixture of both antenatally diagnosed and intraoperatively encountered (19%) abnormally adherent placentas. However, when the intraoperatively diagnosed patients were removed, there continued to be no difference in the prespecified primary outcomes.

BCs and Embolization

As with OBCs, there are many case reports supporting the use of embolization in the management of abnormal placentation. In some instances, embolization was used not only to stem blood loss at the time of hysterectomy but also as part of a strategy to preserve the uterus. Some studies have attempted to evaluate the effects of arterial embolization following OBCs in preparation for hysterectomy. Similar to data on OBCs, there are a conflicting and limited number of studies with an appropriate control group investigating arterial embolization prior to planned hysterectomy. Bodner et al. evaluated 28 consecutive subjects, six of whom received BCs plus embolization compared with 22 subjects who underwent hysterectomy alone and noted no differences in mean estimated blood loss (2.8 vs. 2.6 L; $p = 0.40$), volume of replaced blood products (6.5 vs. 6.3 units; $p = 0.47$), or operating room (OR) time (338 vs. 228 minutes; $p = 0.052$).[13]

In contrast, Angstmann et al. performed a staged-embolization hysterectomy protocol on eight subjects compared with 18 controls and reported benefits of embolization.[14] In this trial, patients were identified with abnormal placentas and on the day of delivery had femoral sheath placement followed by BCs in the IR suite. The patients were then transferred to the OR where a cesarean delivery was performed. If the patient was stable following delivery of the infant, the patient was then transferred to the IR suite and embolized before proceeding with hysterectomy. These cases were compared with patients who underwent hysterectomy alone, some of whom were *not stable* enough for the embolization procedure. The authors did not clearly delineate why some patients were embolized and others were not. These findings noted that embolized subjects had less mean blood loss (553 vs. 4517 mL; $p = 0.0001$) and units transfused (0.5 vs. 7.9 units; $p = 0.0013$). However, there are concerns with the selection of the control group; for example, the use of subjects who were not stable for the embolization portion of the protocol implies that women without embolization may have had more severe disease. This introduces considerable bias and skews the comparison in favor of embolization.

Clearly, the lack of well-designed, randomized prospective studies is the most conspicuous piece of the puzzle missing in evaluating the effectiveness of the interventional procedures. Recently, Salim et al.[15] published a randomized control trial of pre-cesarean prophylactic BCs for suspected placenta accreta. They prospectively randomized 27 women with suspected placenta accreta to either preoperative prophylactic BCs or to a control group. They found no difference between groups in any of the measured endpoints including mean number of PRBC units transfused or in calculated blood loss. Further, two women receiving BCs had reversible adverse effects (leg pain and weakness [unclear etiology] and one case of reversible buttock pain). Unfortunately, not all patients received the same surgical procedure of hysterectomy, as conservative management was an option. In fact, fewer than half of the women had hysterectomies performed initially (six out of thirteen in the treatment and seven out of fourteen in the control group). Consequently, this study was severely underpowered to be able to assess the benefit or lack of benefit with BCs in patients with placenta accreta.

In its absence, retrospective studies with comparison groups represent the only available data. The difficulty in using data from these studies is inherent in their nature—lack of randomization, multiple confounding variables, and introduction of bias. In the studies that failed to demonstrate benefit, a valid criticism is that BCs were placed in subjects with more ominous appearing placentas, thus preventing greater blood loss but obscuring the actual advantage (selection bias). In Ballas et al., where OBCs actually demonstrated benefit, the inclusion of intraoperatively diagnosed accretas implied that these cases lacked the preparation or hemodynamic stability the opposing group possessed. Similarly, in the embolization studies by Angstmann et al., the positive findings noted in their study could be a reflection of the differing characteristics of the groups instead of the studied interventions.

Another plausible explanation for failure to observe benefit from OBCs could be attributed to the timing of when they are deployed. Routine inflation of catheters following delivery of the infant could lead to the establishment of substantial collateral circulation from the network of surrounding vessels diverting blood flow more distally. Angiographic studies of pregnant patients undergoing internal iliac artery ligation have identified branches of the lumbar, sacral, rectal, femoral, and even internal thoracic arteries as the origin of collateral circulation, preventing pelvic ischemia. Strategies such as timing of OBC deployment and placement have been utilized in an effort to avoid development of collateral blood flow. Hull et al. noted that timing of balloon deployment has a critical role in the avoidance of establishing collateral circulation, thus curtailing significant blood loss.[16] Specifically, the OBCs are inflated only when "torrential hemorrhage" is encountered; routine deployment following delivery may actually be "counter-productive." The implication of this hypothesis is that the reason for the lack of perceived benefit noted in the negative trials is the immediate deployment of OBCs. More strategic inflation during the precarious points of surgery may avert engorged collateral vasculature, therefore averting greater blood loss. This technique of delayed inflation was performed only in the Ballas et al. trial, which found benefit in OBCs.

Another factor to consider is the site of placement of the OBCs. Placement of the OBCs more proximally in the vasculature tree would avoid the formation of collateral blood flow, but at the potential expense of limb ischemia (Figure 8.3). Studies to date have evaluated placement in branches of the anterior division of the internal iliacs, thus providing focused occlusion of the uterine blood flow. While there have been case reports of anecdotal success with placing OBCs in more proximal vasculature such as the aorta or common iliac arteries, one series which focused primarily on percretas noted continued significant blood loss and questionable efficacy of more proximally placed OBCs for controlling hemorrhage.[17] Matsubara et al. modified their technique to occlude the common iliac artery instead of the internal iliac arteries following observations of inadequate control of bleeding with the internal iliac occlusion technique.[18] To date, there have been no prospective randomized studies evaluating proximal placement of OBCs.

Perhaps the most significant factor contributing to the inability to demonstrate benefit from interventional procedures may come from the heterogeneity of abnormal placentation. This is a concept first demonstrated by Cali et al. who noted that the potential benefits of OBCs were lost when placenta percretas were selected out. The implication of this finding suggests that the performance of a cesarean hysterectomy for any indication is subject to significant blood loss. The presence of less invasive placentas, such as accretas and possibly incretas, may not contribute to substantially more blood loss than the performance of hysterectomy alone. Thus, the use of OBCs could theoretically have a clinically negligible benefit. However, in cases of more extensively invasive placentas, where blood loss tends to be significant, the use of OBCs may have a favorable effect on total blood loss. With the exception of Cali et al., all studies evaluated the effects of OBCs on all types of abnormally adherent placenta as a group, with no subanalysis or stratification by severity of placental pathology. The implication of this argument highlights the need for a presurgical classification of abnormally adherent placentas so that appropriate comparisons are made.

It would appear that the use of OBCs should be considered experimental with no clear proof of efficacy for any particular form of abnormal placentation. Further, there have been unfortunate complications

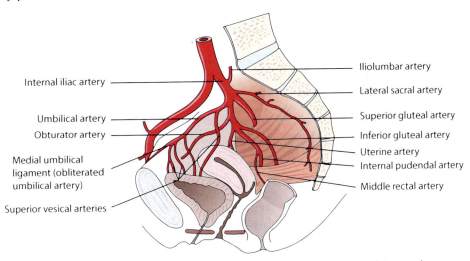

FIGURE 8.3 Branches of the internal iliac artery in the female.

with IR procedures. However, perhaps in specific circumstances, in a setting of highly concerning evidence of severely abnormal placentation such as suspected percreta, the use of OBCs should be considered. Finally, for the patient who has had uterine conservation surgery following the use of either or both OBCs and uterine artery embolization for abnormal placentation, the long-term health issues with regard to menstrual function, fertility, and overall health remain unclear.

REFERENCES

1. Miller DA, Chollet JA, Goodwin TM. Clinical risk factors for placenta previa-placenta accreta. *Am J Obstet Gynecol.* 1997;177(1):210–214.
2. Brown BJ, Heaston DK, Poulson AM, Gabert HA, Mineau DE, Miller FJ Jr. Uncontrollable postpartum bleeding: A new approach to hemostasis through angiographic arterial embolization. *Obstet Gynecol.* 1979;54:361–365.
3. Mitty HA, Sterling KM, Alvarez M, Gendler R. Obstetric hemorrhage: Prophylactic and emergency arterial catheterization and embolotherapy. *Radiology.* 1993;188:183–187.
4. Alanis M, Hurst BS, Marshburn PB, Matthews ML. Conservative management of placenta increta with selective arterial embolization preserves future fertility and results in a favorable outcome in subsequent pregnancies. *Fertil Steril.* 2006;86:1514e3–1514e7.
5. Carnevale FC, Kondo MM, De Oliveira Sousa W Jr., et al. Perioperative temporary occlusion of the internal iliac arteries as prophylaxis in cesarean section at risk of hemorrhage in placenta accreta. *Cardiovasc Intervent Radiol.* 2011;34:758–764.
6. Thon S, McLintic A, Wagner Y. Prophylactic endovascular placement of internal iliac occlusion balloon catheters in parturients with placenta accreta: A retrospective case series. *Int J Obstet Anesth.* 2011;20:64–70.
7. Tan CH, Tay KH, Sheah K, Kwek K, Wong K, Tan HK, Tan BS. Perioperative endovascular internal iliac artery occlusion balloon placement in management of placenta accreta. *Am J Roentgenol.* 2007;189(5):1158–1163.
8. Ballas J, Hull AD, Saenz C, et al. Preoperative intravascular balloon catheters and surgical outcomes in pregnancies complicated by placenta accreta: A management paradox. *Am J Obstet Gynecol.* 2012;207(3):e1–5.
9. Cali G, Forlani F, Giambanco L. Prophylactic use of intravascular balloon catheters in women with placenta accreta, increta and percreta. *Eur J Obstet Gynecol Reprod Biol.* 2014;179:36–41.
10. Levine, AB, Kuhlman K, Bonn J. Placenta accreta: Comparison of cases managed with and without pelvic artery balloon catheters. *J Matern Fetal Med.* 1999;8(4):173–176.
11. Tan, CH, Tay KH, Sheah K, et al. Perioperative endovascular internal iliac artery occlusion balloon placement in management of placenta accreta. *AJR Am J Roentgenol.* 2007;189(5): 1158–1163.
12. Shrivastava V, Nageotte MP, Major C, Haydon M, Wing D. Case-control comparison of cesarean hysterectomy with and without prophylactic placement of intravascular balloon catheters for placenta accreta. *Am J Obstet Gynecol.* 2007;197(4):402 e1–5.
13. Bodner LJ, Nosher JL, Gribbin C, Siegel RL, Beale S. Balloon-assisted occlusion of the internal iliac arteries in patients with placenta accreta/percreta. *Cardiovasc Intervent Radiol.* 2006;29(3):354–361.
14. Angstmann T, Gard G, Harington T, Ward E, Thomson A, Giles W. Surgical management of placenta accreta: A cohort series and suggested approach. *Am J Obstet Gynecol.* 2010;202(1):38 e1–9.
15. Salim R, Chulski A, Romano S, Garmi G, Rudin M, Shalev E. Precesarean prophylatic balloon catheters for suspected placenta accreta. *Obstet Gynecol.* 2015;126:1022–1028.
16. Hull, AD, Resnik R. Placenta accreta and postpartum hemorrhage. *Clin Obstet Gynecol.* 2010;53(1):228–236.
17. Clausen C, Stensballe J, Albrechtsen CK, Hansen MA, Lonn L, Langhoff-Roos J. Balloon occlusion of the internal iliac arteries in the multidisciplinary management of placenta percreta. *Acta Obstet Gynecol Scand.* 2013;92(4):386–391.
18. Matsubara S, Yano H, Ohkuchi A, Kuwata T, Usui R, Suzuki M. Important surgical measures and techniques at cesarean hysterectomy for placenta previa accreta. *Acta Obstet Gynecol Scand.* 2013;92(4):372–377.
19. Penning S, Roy K, Garite TJ, et al. The efficacy of hypogastric artery occlusion via balloon catheters for cesarean hysterectomy. *Am J Obstet Gynecol.* 2001;185(6):S109.

9

Center of Excellence for Morbidly Adherent Placenta

Karin A. Fox, Alireza A. Shamshirsaz, and Michael A. Belfort

CONTENTS

> Excellence is an art won by training and habituation. We are what we repeatedly do. Excellence therefore is not an act, but a habit.
>
> **—Aristotle**

Introduction

As described in previous chapters, morbidly adherent placenta (MAP), including the spectrum of placenta accreta, increta, and percreta, encompasses some of the most challenging alterations of the uteroplacental unit encountered in obstetrics. Management of MAP is equally complex. In addition to the usual changes in maternal physiology that occur during pregnancy, there is often distorted anatomy due to placental invasion and neovascularization that varies in degree and location from patient to patient. The potential for torrential bleeding demands a high level of planning and organization, surgical and procedural skill, and detailed, multidisciplinary attention to the timing of surgery, maintenance (or recovery) of hemodynamic stability, integrity of the coagulation system, and intensive care support.

What Is a "Center of Excellence"?

The term "Center of Excellence" (CoE) is used across multiple professions, ranging from corporate and government arenas to health care and academia. Although individual organizations structure and focus their respective CoEs differently, the following quotation in our opinion most closely defines the concept: "A center of excellence is a team, a shared facility or an entity that provides leadership, best practices, research, support and/or training for a focus area."[1]

On July 30, 1965, Lyndon B. Johnson signed into law Title XVIII and Title XIX of the Social Security Act, effectively creating Medicare and Medicaid to ensure health care access for citizens over the age of 65 and people getting cash assistance. Since then, the scope and roles of the Center for Medicare and Medicaid Services (CMS) have expanded greatly. Part of the mission of the CMS is to provide high-quality health care to approximately 37.2 million participants. In an effort to improve care in the early 1990s, the CMS designated certain facilities as "Centers of Excellence" for various complex procedures, including cardiac bypass, orthopedic surgery, and bariatric surgeries. Currently, such centers are officially designated "approved facilities," but are commonly referred to as CoEs in the medical literature. CMS limited reimbursement to approved facilities, "with the stipulation that the facilities providing these services meet certain criteria," one of which is that they "meet the minimum standards to ensure the safety of beneficiaries receiving these services in order to be considered as a provider with the ability and expertise to perform the procedure."[2] A substantial amount of information regarding outcomes, processes, and protocols has become available that allows comparison with non-participating centers (i.e., those servicing privately insured patients), with mixed results.[3–8]

The CMS has not designated "approved facilities" for diagnosis and management of placenta accreta. In decades past, placenta accreta was considered relatively rare. Data regarding best practices and standards of care for MAP continue to evolve in response to a rising incidence of the disease, and data are accumulating to show that outcomes in specialized units managing placenta accreta are better than in "standard" facilities. While we do not necessarily advocate for mandated credentialing for CoE designation for purposes of CMS reimbursement, we suggest (and highlight with peer-reviewed evidence) that women with MAP are best managed in a center designed for this purpose. In this chapter, we outline the resources essential to building a comprehensive, highly functional, multidisciplinary team to optimize the care of women with MAP and present the case for defining a CoE as one that can objectively demonstrate having robust systems in place and an experienced team that not only provides excellent care but that also guides improvement in practice through ongoing educational programs and clinical, scientific, and quality research.

Surgical management of patients with MAP by an experienced, multidisciplinary team in a tertiary center reduces the need for massive transfusion, second surgery, or a composite morbidity when compared with women delivered in traditional settings.[9] While hysterectomy following cesarean without attempts to remove the placenta is widely accepted as one form of definitive management,[10,11] conservative management using procedures designed to avoid hysterectomy has been popularized in Europe and is increasingly being practiced with varying degrees of success.[12–17] The major risks of leaving the uterus in situ include hemorrhage, disseminated intravascular coagulopathy (DIC), intrauterine infection, sepsis, prolonged recovery, and the need for delayed or emergent hysterectomy.[18] Because these may arise unpredictably, in some cases as late as 9 months postpartum,[14,19,20] it is our opinion that conservative management should be undertaken by teams experienced in recognition and management of potential complications, with close surveillance, and only when definitive surgery is not safe or feasible.

What Constitutes a Multidisciplinary Team for Placenta Accreta Care?

The criteria suggested[20] for MAP by CoE patient care are given in Table 9.1.

Ideal management of placenta accreta begins in the antenatal period with early, accurate identification of findings on antenatal imaging, most commonly ultrasound, with magnetic resonance imaging (MRI) as an adjunctive imaging modality.[21,22] Surgery in patients who had prenatal diagnosis of MAP is associated with lower estimated blood loss and lower total volume of transfusion at the time of delivery than in those who had intrapartum diagnosis, without significant increases in neonatal morbidity.[21,23]

In large population-based studies, which include patients screened in both large academic centers and in community clinics, antenatal diagnosis only occurs in approximately 50% of cases.[24,25] The sensitivity and specificity of antenatal diagnosis of MAP in studies reported from large, tertiary referral centers suggests a higher sensitivity (ultrasound: 70%–100% and MRI: 86%–96%) and specificity (ultrasound: 37%–94% and MRI: 77%–88%).[26–28]

We recommend referral for specialized imaging for patients with prior cesarean deliveries or prior uterine surgeries (especially multiple cesareans), placenta previa, history of endometrial ablation prior to pregnancy, and first- or second-trimester bleeding in the presence of other accreta risk factors. Referral is also recommended any time initial screening ultrasound suggests an abnormality (abnormal placental appearance, abnormal uterine shape, increased vascularity of the myometrial wall or current or prior cesarean scar, ectopic pregnancy).[29] Use of a diagnostic checklist may alert sonographers and imaging experts to significant risk factors and should prompt closer inspection of the placenta. In addition, such a

TABLE 9.1

Suggested Criteria

---

1. Multidisciplinary Physician Team (with 24-hour availability)
   a. Experienced clinician (maternal–fetal medicine [MFM] or generalist obstetrician/gynecologist [ob/gyn]) with experience in managing all aspects of morbidly adherent placenta (MAP), and in particular the unique techniques required in MAP surgery
   b. Imaging experts (2D and 3D/color Doppler ultrasound and magnetic resonance imaging [MRI])
   c. Pelvic surgeon (i.e., gynecologic oncologist or urogynecologist)
   d. Urologist
   e. Trauma or vascular surgeon
   f. Neonatologist
2. Intensive care unit (ICU) and facilities
   a. Surgical or medical ICU with 24-hour availability of intensive care specialists
   b. Neonatal ICU with support appropriate for the gestational age of the neonate
3. Interventional radiology team
   a. Ideally capable of performing embolization or intravascular balloon
   b. Placement in the operating room (OR) rather than a separate radiology suite
4. Blood bank/transfusion medicine services
   a. Massive transfusion capabilities
   b. Cell saver and perfusionist staff qualified to set up and run the machine
   c. Experience with and availability of alternative blood products
   d. Transfusion medicine specialists or blood bank pathologists
5. Support staff experienced or trained in care of patients with MAP
   a. Circulating and floor nurses
   b. Surgical technicians
   c. Physical therapy/occupational therapist
   d. Social work and/or psychiatrist/psychologist

Source: Adapted from Silver RM et al., *Am J Obstet Gynecol,* 212(5), 561–568, 2014.

checklist may help identify patients for whom MRI may be useful. A full discussion of antenatal imaging is beyond the scope of this chapter but can be found in Chapters 3 and 4.

The psychological and social impact of placenta accreta has yet to be fully elucidated; however, studies suggest that traumatic birth experiences increase a woman's risk for postpartum depression or posttraumatic stress disorder.[30] Birth experiences, both positive and negative, persist over a 5-year period.[31] Providing a patient adequate time to establish care in a CoE provides the opportunity to develop a relationship with the care team, which fosters trust, as well as emotional and psychological support. This allows the patient to coordinate time away from work and family as needed, to consult with individual multidisciplinary team specialists, tour the neonatal intensive care unit ICU when possible, and ask questions regarding her care.

Antenatal diagnosis and early referral allow the team to develop an individualized plan of care, taking into consideration each individual's obstetrical history, current pregnancy course, potential medical comorbidities, and social circumstances. In general, delivery between 34 and 35 weeks gestation is advised to balance the risk of maternal bleeding against neonatal prematurity[32,33]; however, earlier delivery is warranted in the setting of active bleeding and in women with preterm premature rupture of membranes or increasing uterine activity.[34] Conversely, some patients who remain very stable throughout pregnancy with no bleeding and no preterm contractions may be able to safely deliver at 36 weeks gestation.[35]

At our center, we routinely admit patients to the antepartum unit 5–7 days prior to a scheduled cesarean hysterectomy to allow for multidisciplinary consultation and antenatal corticosteroid administration. Earlier admission is recommended whenever patients have recurrent or significant bleeding, regular uterine contractions, or rupture of membranes. In some cases, a patient may live in a location that would not allow rapid, safe comprehensive management in the event of an emergency, and in this event it seems reasonable to house patients in domiciliary care or intermediate care close to or within the hospital for some time prior to delivery. In our patients with MAP who delivered between January 2013 and December 2015, approximately 50% of patients required delivery prior to their planned date of delivery due to contractions, bleeding, or other maternal or fetal indication, consistent with other cohorts.[34,35] This underscores the importance of counseling patients about signs and symptoms of labor and staying near a hospital with appropriate facilities as delivery nears.

The cornerstones of effective teamwork are (1) clear communication between all team members and (2) dedication toward responding to the call for service, especially in cases of emergency or unanticipated delivery. By developing systems of communication and notification, team members from all specialties and subspecialties can be quickly and efficiently apprised of upcoming cases, new admissions, and the need for emergent surgical support. At our facility, a clinical nurse coordinator screens all referrals and schedules an initial visit for imaging and consultation with a maternal–fetal medicine (MFM) provider. Once MAP is substantively confirmed by imaging, or whenever the clinical suspicion remains sufficiently high (for example, in a gravida 6 with five prior cesarean sections and placenta previa, even in the absence of clear imaging findings), the patient is counseled about MAP and is given written information for her own reference and to facilitate discussion with family members. A delivery date is set, usually between 34 and 35 weeks gestation, and an operating room (OR) in our dedicated obstetrician/gynecologist (ob/gyn) OR suite is reserved during weekly scheduled block time for MAP cases. Should this block time remain unscheduled 2 weeks prior to the date, the OR time slots are opened to other providers for scheduled cesarean deliveries. This minimizes disruption of previously scheduled cases and facilitates planning for the multidisciplinary surgeons.

Some centers discuss pending cases at regularly scheduled multidisciplinary meetings to review imaging, pertinent patient history, and discuss scheduling and planning. Because of our individual circumstances, we utilize asynchronous communication to allow team members the flexibility to review cases as their schedules allow. All pending cases are maintained on a list within the electronic medical record, which is shared among all MAP team members and support staff. Within each record there is a "snapshot" note that includes scheduled dates of admission and surgery, contact information, and links to imaging and medical and surgical history. Weekly or biweekly notification of upcoming cases is circulated by secure e-mail, with the expectation that members from each respective surgical service will respond with the name of the surgeon(s) who will be present for the case.

To cover unscheduled or emergent cases, we provide all floors with a call schedule, listing names and phone numbers of physicians available each night and weekend. Advanced preparation of such a schedule helps ensure complete coverage and helps us avoid under- or unstaffed intervals. This schedule is made available electronically to all physicians and nursing personnel along with electronic access to a standardized combined consent form, checklists, and workflow algorithms.

Upon admission, a standardized order set is used to prompt providers to keep typed and cross-matched blood on hold, to consult team services, and to administer corticosteroids and magnesium sulfate for neuroprotection, when appropriate. The patient's nurse is expected to complete a paper checklist (Figure 9.1) that remains on the patient's paper chart. This checklist can be readily accessed in case of electronic system downtime or failure, or while transporting a patient in the event of an emergency. At least one member of the MAP team sees the patient daily from the time of admission until discharge.

Should a patient begin to bleed, contract, or have other indications for delivery, we utilize a "call tree" approach. Rather than have one person call in every team member, notification is initiated and performed by ancillary personnel (house supervisor). This frees the bedside nurse and/or attending physician to remain at the bedside to work to stabilize or mobilize the patient. The house supervisor will then contact the "first call" MFM team member, who then calls the gynecologic oncologist, urologist, and interventional radiologist, and gives a report. Simultaneously, the house supervisor alerts the OR staff, in-house anesthesiology team, and blood bank personnel who can begin setting up the OR, assessing the patient, and ensuring that blood and blood products are ready, in preparation for possible activation of the massive transfusion protocol. The house supervisor then reports back to the MFM with the anticipated "rollback" time to the OR. Likewise, the MFM physician updates the house supervisor with estimated times of arrival for team members. The house supervisor or his or her designee will also notify the neonatal ICU. In cases of true emergency, when a patient is actively bleeding, this process may be expedited by activating an emergency response button that is stationed in each room. Other facilities may have an overhead page code or emergency page that alerts all key team members to go directly to the patient's

Placenta Accreta Safety Checklist		
Antepartum and BPR Pre-Surgical Checklist		**OR Pre- and Intra-Operative Checklist**

Consults	**Consents**	**Anesthesiology**
☐ MFM	☐ Cesarean section	☐ Antibiotic prophylaxis
_____	☐ Hysterectomy	☐ Methergine in OR
☐ GYN oncologist	☐ Cystoscopy with bilateral stent placement	☐ Hemabate in OR
_____	☐ Epidural/spinal/general	☐ Misoprostil in OR
☐ Urology	☐ Arterial line	☐ Normothermia measures
_____	☐ Central line	
☐ Anesthesiology		
☐ Intensive care		
☐ Interventional radiology		
Laboratory		**Risk of Blood Loss (>1000mL)**
Hemoglobin _____ Hematocrit _____		☐ Blood in OR (4 units PRBCs; 4 units FFP; 4 and 4 in blood bank)
☐ Prenatal labs		
☐ Type and cross within last 72 hours		☐ Cell saver (equipment and personnel)
☐ Other:		
Blood Bank Notified: _____ (date)		**Nursing**
☐ 4 Units PRBCs and FFP to OR		☐ VTE prophylaxis: SCDs on
		☐ EFM during/after epidural/spinal
Nursing		**Surgical specialties**
☐ Patient allergies: _____ /banded _____		*MFM and GYN-Oncology*
☐ Admission navigator complete		☐ Cesarean section/hysterectomy
☐ Newborn identification to OR		*Urology*
☐ EFM in BPR		☐ Instruments, equipment, and supplies
☐ VTE prophylaxis: SCDs on		*Interventional Radiology*
		☐ On stand-by
		☐ Instruments, equipment, and supplies
Medications		**Other equipment/supplies requested by surgeon**
☐ Pre-op anesthesia		☐
☐ Antibiotic to OR		☐
☐ **Pre-brief completed**		**Patient sticker**

FIGURE 9.1 Placenta accreta safety checklist. MFM, maternal–fetal medicine; GYN, gynecologic; PRBCs, packed red blood cells; FFP, fresh frozen plasma; EFM, electronic fetal monitoring; VTE, venous thromboembolism; SCD, sequential compression device; OR, operating room.

room for assessment and planning. The checklist (Figure 9.1) again helps remind the team of essential safety steps.

Education and Outreach

Given that evidence suggests that centers with the appropriate resources and highly experienced teams have the best outcomes, we believe that those medical systems participating in (hospitals and insurance payers), or responsible for providing or overseeing (federal and state legislators) such care have an imperative to develop teams and ensure that facilities meet the clinical demands of the future. Although the incidence of MAP is rising, it remains relatively rare, with an estimated incidence between 1 in 533 and 1 in 1200 pregnancies. In comparison, other high-risk perinatal conditions such as preeclampsia or diabetes occur in approximately 5%–10% of all pregnancies.[36,37] Identification and appropriate management of patients with conditions that occur rarely, but are of the highest risk, are contingent upon early recognition of the disease and access to appropriate care. Many CoEs are academic referral centers, which provide an opportunity for students, residents, and junior faculty to gain exposure to patients with MAP. It is reasonable to question whether residents and fellows should continue to participate in long, complex percreta cases, where experts may need to "take over" part of the surgery, especially in the setting of duty-hour limitations. One argument is that trainees may be better served performing a larger number of routine cesarean deliveries and hysterectomies rather than participate partially or marginally in such complex cases. The majority of ob/gyn residents in training will not work in a large tertiary care center, and they may not care for women with MAP. We argue that trainee participation in the care and management of MAP is not only enriching but also essential. The ability to recognize the MAP antenatally or even after opening the abdomen, but prior to hysterotomy, may be life-saving if it allows safe transfer of the patient to an appropriate center. The ability to instantly recognize a placenta accreta or increta simply by looking at the morphology of the lower uterine segment (often obscured by adherent bladder or omentum) is something that only comes with experience. The technique for a safe cesarean section in a patient with placenta percreta (exteriorized uterus, minimal blood loss techniques, and fundal or posterior hysterotomy) is not intuitive, and experience is invaluable in learning to do it. Trainee involvement also prompts understanding of the considerable morbidity of MAP as well as reflection and the opportunity for more in-depth discussion. We have had more than one resident mention in the OR, "What should do if I see this in the OR with one of my patients after I graduate?" Finally, direct involvement managing patients in the postpartum period exposes learners to complex postoperative care that translates to care for any postoperative patient, including, but not limited to, management of occult hemorrhage, urinary tract injury, ileus or small bowel obstruction, and management of the patient in an ICU.

Education and outreach not only involve physician trainees but the entire multidisciplinary team. An anesthesiology colleague recently commented that the volume of MAP cases at our center, our multidisciplinary approach, and our coordinated simulation training have all led to an increased familiarity among the nursing and support staff with regard to recognition of hypovolemia, implementation of our massive transfusion, and rapid response protocols. Moreover, this familiarity has translated into improved efficiency in their response to obstetrical hemorrhage from causes other than MAP.

Patient and family education and outreach are central components of patient care. It is striking how few patients or their families have heard of placenta accreta prior to their index pregnancy. This will likely change as the incidence of MAP rises and the ability of former patients and patient advocacy groups gain traction through organized outreach and social media venues. In the United States and other high-resource settings, the incidence of maternal mortality and severe morbidity has decreased dramatically in the last century, and an individual woman's perception of risk regarding pregnancy and delivery is likely much different than that of our grandmothers and great-grandmothers or women in low-resource settings where access to care and safe surgical practices are unavailable. Our role as clinicians is to provide accurate, balanced, individualized and evidence-based advice to our patients. This requires having the requisite venues and personnel/materials to allow full discussion of imaging findings, risks of the condition itself, and the risks and benefits of the recommended treatment plan. There should also be ample time to allow the patient and her family to ask and receive answers to their questions. Often an ongoing conversation that occurs over several visits is required. There is limited evidence suggesting that women with high-risk conditions and women who perceive their deliveries as traumatic may be impacted negatively both emotionally and/or psychologically. Further studies are required to confirm this association and to determine whether interventions such as perinatal counseling or postpartum debriefing can ameliorate this impact.

Research and Quality Improvement

Tertiary care centers have long upheld the mission not only to care for patients most in need and teach the next generation of clinicians, but also to advance scientific knowledge about disease and health through research. Currently, a majority of evidence regarding MAP is based on expert opinion or single-center, retrospective studies. CoEs for MAP should ideally provide the infrastructure for research into the etiology and pathologic mechanisms of abnormal placental invasion, as well as for collaborative clinical and translational research. Such infrastructure includes collaboration between the above-mentioned multidisciplinary services, support for grant preparation and management, the appropriate internal or external institutional review boards to ensure the protection of human research participants, and staff support to conduct research in a timely, ethical manner.

The level of research support and focus will likely vary between centers, depending upon patient populations and volumes seen at each facility, faculty/clinician areas of expertise, local laboratory expertise, and research core availability. No matter the size or scope of the center, active participation in research should be a priority. For example, a smaller center with limited basic science laboratory support may still collaborate with larger centers or networks to implement and enter their data into a network database/registry that enables the reliable collation of demographic variables, medical and surgical history, and short- and long-term outcomes, including physical and psychosocial outcomes and long-term effects of MAP on maternal and child health. While other centers may be better equipped to perform sophisticated sample analysis for molecular marker or genetic studies, each participating center can still contribute to the greater collective body of evidence.

To ensure that research studies are, generalizable, and appropriately powered, a collaborative research approach between CoEs may be required. A number of large, well-powered, multicenter studies have arisen within the field of MFM in the last three decades, especially since the establishment of the Maternal–Fetal Medicine Units (MFMU) Network in 1986 and the Obstetric-Fetal Pharmacology Research Unit (OPRU) Network in 2004, both supported by the Eunice Kennedy Shriver National Institute of Child Health and Human Development (NICHD). National surveillance groups such as the United Kingdom Obstetrical Surveillance System (UKOSS) from the National Perinatal Epidemiology Unit (NPEU) established in 1978 in Oxford, the US Centers for Disease Control (CDC) Pregnancy Risk Assessment Monitoring System (PRAMS) developed in 1987, or the Swedish Medical Birth Register founded in 1973 provide population-level data regarding trends and outcomes. In order to adequately develop generalizable, standardized, and best practice methodologies for the management of MAP, given its relatively low incidence combined with multiple different management protocols currently used, multicenter collaboration with standard protocols seems the best approach. Only by sharing data regarding diagnosis, treatment approaches, and outcomes can we meaningfully answer some of the questions regarding treatment modality, genetic predisposition, and pathophysiology. Such studies have the potential to impact not only the science behind MAP but also public health policy with regard to maternal morbidity and mortality.

The European Working Group on Abnormally Invasive Placenta (EW-AIP, www.ew-aip.org) is an international, multicenter group dedicated to developing such collaborations within Europe. Its aim is to develop a registry specific to abnormally invasive placentation and thereby produce and publish large cohort studies. Such a consortium has also been under development in the United States, with the aim to provide a large, multicenter database and biospecimen bank for large, cohort, and translational research studies. The specimen bank comprises samples of maternal serum, plasma, cord blood, and amniotic fluid when available. Placental and uterine sample collection is planned from areas with normal, marginal, and invasive placental tissue after delivery and hysterectomy to allow study of changes within the placenta and adjacent myometrium at the cellular and molecular levels.

Innovation is integral to a research CoE in MAP. Development and use of cutting-edge technology may play an important role in improving diagnosis as well as therapeutic approaches. The use of 3D Doppler ultrasound and MRI to identify placenta percreta are prime examples of how innovative use of available technology may refine diagnosis, and it is probable that other innovations will also improve treatment.

An essential component of care that can (and must) be promoted at any CoE is quality improvement. Examples may include projects designed to reduce the time from referral to initial consultation or those that aim to reduce the time from decision for urgent delivery to initiation of moving the patient to the OR. Even smaller centers that may not be poised to engage as robustly in scientific research can contribute locally and regionally through quality improvement endeavors.

Clinical Culture and Prevention

Finally, although CoEs for MAP must focus on treatment and management, such centers are in a unique position to promote strategies to prevent patients from developing MAP. As cesarean delivery remains a major risk factor for MAP, it follows that these CoEs work in concert with the Consortium for Safe Labor, the NICHD, and the American College of Obstetricians and Gynecologists to reduce the cesarean delivery rate. While effecting cultural change in medicine may be difficult, it is not impossible, and our commitment to the safety of our patients and their families must remain the highest priority in our care. In the words of Hippocrates, our goal is to "make a habit of two things—to help, or at least, to do no harm."

REFERENCES

1. Center of Excellence, Wikipedia.com. https://en.wikipedia.org/wiki/Center_of_excellence#cite _note-Mark 2010-1.
2. Medicare Approved Facilities/Trials/Registries CMS.gov: Center for Medicare and Medicaid Services. January 31, 2016. Available at: https://www.cms.gov/Medicare/Medicare-General-Information/Medicare ApprovedFacilitie/. Accessed on May 9, 2014.
3. Doumouras AG, Saleh F, Hong D. 30-Day readmission after bariatric surgery in a publicly funded regionalized center of excellence system. *Surg Endosc.* 2015;30(5):2066–2072.
4. Doumouras AG, Saleh F, Tarride JE, Hong D. A population-based analysis of the drivers of short-term costs after bariatric surgery within a publicly funded regionalized center of excellence system. *Surg Obes Relat Dis.* 2016;12(5):1023–1031.
5. Doumouras AG, Saleh F, Gmora S, Anvari M, Hong D. Regional variations in the public delivery of bariatric surgery: An evaluation of the center of excellence model. *Ann Surg.* 2016;263(2):306–311.
6. Abdelgawad M, De Angelis F, Iossa A, Rizzello M, Cavallaro G, Silecchia G. Management of complications and outcomes after revisional bariatric surgery: 3-year experience at a bariatric center of excellence. *Obes Surg.* 2016;26(9):2144–2149.
7. Scally CP, Shih T, Thumma JR, Dimick JB. Impact of a national bariatric surgery center of excellence program on medicare expenditures. *J Gastrointest Surg.* 2016;20(4):708–714.
8. Mehrotra A, Sloss EM, Hussey PS, Adams JL, Lovejoy S, SooHoo NF. Evaluation of a center of excellence program for spine surgery. *Med Care.* 2013;51(8):748–757.
9. Eller AG, Bennett MA, Sharshiner M, et al. Maternal morbidity in cases of placenta accreta managed by a multidisciplinary care team compared with standard obstetric care. *Obstet Gynecol.* 2011; 117(2 Pt 1):331–337.
10. Practice CoO. Committee opinion no. 529: Placenta accreta. *Obstet Gynecol.* 2012;120(1):207–211.
11. Allahdin S, Voigt S, Htwe TT. Management of placenta praevia and accreta. *J Obstet Gynaecol.* 2011;31(1):1–6.
12. Chandraharan E, Rao S, Belli AM, Arulkumaran S. The Triple-P procedure as a conservative surgical alternative to peripartum hysterectomy for placenta percreta. *Int J Gynaecol Obstet.* 2012;117(2):191–194.
13. Alanis M, Hurst BS, Marshburn PB, Matthews ML. Conservative management of placenta increta with selective arterial embolization preserves future fertility and results in a favorable outcome in subsequent pregnancies. *Fertil Steril.* 2006;86(5):1514. e3–7.
14. Clausen C, Lonn L, Langhoff-Roos J. Management of placenta percreta: A review of published cases. *Acta Obstet Gynecol Scand.* 2014;93(2):138–143.
15. Kayem G, Davy C, Goffinet F, Thomas C, Clement D, Cabrol D. Conservative versus extirpative management in cases of placenta accreta. *Obstet Gynecol.* 2004;104(3):531–536.
16. Sentilhes L, Kayem G, Ambroselli C, et al. Fertility and pregnancy outcomes following conservative treatment for placenta accreta. *Hum Reprod.* 2010;25(11):2803–2810.
17. Sentilhes L, Ambroselli C, Kayem G, et al. Maternal outcome after conservative treatment of placenta accreta. *Obstet Gynecol.* 2010;115(3):526–534.
18. Fox KA, Shamshirsaz AA, Carusi D, et al. Conservative management of morbidly adherent placenta: Expert review. *Am J Obstet Gynecol.* 2015; 213(6):755–760.
19. Kayem G, Davy C, Goffinet F, Thomas C, Clément D, Cabrol D. Conservative versus extirpative management in cases of placenta accreta. *Obstet Gynecol.* 2004;104(3):531–536.
20. Roulot A, Barranger E, Morel O, Soyer P, Hequet D. [Two- and three-dimensional power Doppler ultrasound in the follow-up of placenta accreta treated conservatively.]. *J Gynecol Obstet Biol Reprod (Paris).* 2015;44(2):176–183.
21. Warshak CR, Ramos GA, Eskander R, et al. Effect of predelivery diagnosis in 99 consecutive cases of placenta accreta. *Obstet Gynecol.* 2010;115(1):65–69.

22. Warshak CR, Eskander R, Hull AD, et al. Accuracy of ultrasonography and magnetic resonance imaging in the diagnosis of placenta accreta. *Obstet Gynecol.* 2006;108(3 Pt 1):573–581.

23. Tikkanen M, Paavonen J, Loukovaara M, Stefanovic V. Antenatal diagnosis of placenta accreta leads to reduced blood loss. *Acta Obstet Gynecol Scand.* 2011;90(10):1140–1146.

24. Bailit JL, Grobman WA, Rice MM, et al. Morbidly adherent placenta treatments and outcomes. *Obstet Gynecol.* 2015;125(3):683–689.

25. Fitzpatrick KE, Sellers S, Spark P, Kurinczuk JJ, Brocklehurst P, Knight M. The management and outcomes of placenta accreta, increta, and percreta in the UK: A population-based descriptive study. *BJOG.* 2014;121(1):62–70; discussion -1.

26. D'Antonio F, Iacovella C, Palacios-Jaraquemada J, Bruno CH, Manzoli L, Bhide A. Prenatal identification of invasive placentation using magnetic resonance imaging: Systematic review and meta-analysis. *Ultrasound Obstet Gynecol.* 2014;44(1):8–16.

27. Rezk MA, Shawky M. Grey-scale and colour Doppler ultrasound versus magnetic resonance imaging for the prenatal diagnosis of placenta accreta. *J Matern Fetal Neonatal Med.* 2014:1–6.

28. Maher MA, Abdelaziz A, Bazeed MF. Diagnostic accuracy of ultrasound and MRI in the prenatal diagnosis of placenta accreta. *Acta Obstet Gynecol Scand.* 2013;92(9):1017–1022.

29. Silver RM, Fox KA, Barton JR, et al. Center of excellence for placenta accreta. *Am J Obstet Gynecol.* 2015;212(5):561–568.

30. Halperin O, Sarid O, Cwikel J. The influence of childbirth experiences on women's postpartum traumatic stress symptoms: A comparison between Israeli Jewish and Arab women. *Midwifery.* 2015;31(6):625–632.

31. Takehara K, Noguchi M, Shimane T, Misago C. A longitudinal study of women's memories of their childbirth experiences at five years postpartum. *BMC Pregnancy Childbirth.* 2014;14:221.

32. Robinson BK, Grobman WA. Effectiveness of timing strategies for delivery of individuals with placenta previa and accreta. *Obstet Gynecol.* 2010;116(4):835–842.

33. Publications Committee SfM-FM, Belfort MA. Placenta accreta. *Am J Obstet Gynecol.* 2010;203(5):430–439.

34. Bowman ZS, Manuck TA, Eller AG, Simons M, Silver RM. Risk factors for unscheduled delivery in patients with placenta accreta. *Am J Obstet Gynecol.* 2014;210(3):241. e1–6.

35. Rac MW, Wells CE, Twickler DM, Moschos E, McIntire DD, Dashe JS. Placenta accreta and vaginal bleeding according to gestational age at delivery. *Obstet Gynecol.* 2015;125(4):808–813.

36. Committee Opinion Summary No. 638: First-trimester risk assessment for early-onset preeclampsia. *Obstet Gynecol.* 2015;126(3):689.

37. DeSisto CL, Kim SY, Sharma AJ. Prevalence estimates of gestational diabetes mellitus in the United States, pregnancy risk assessment monitoring system (PRAMS), 2007–2010. *Prev Chronic Dis.* 2014;11:E104.

10

Blood Management for Patients with Placenta Accreta

Andra H. James and Evelyn Lockhart

CONTENTS

Background

Approximately 50% of patients with placenta accreta (including increta and percreta) experience postpartum hemorrhage (PPH); of those patients, 20%–95% are transfused.[1-4] Half to three quarters of these transfusions are massive, requiring four or more units of red blood cells (RBCs).[3,5] There are few specific data regarding other blood products, but in one retrospective review of 66 subjects with accreta—95% were transfused with RBCs, 64% received plasma, 23% received cryoprecipitate, and 42% received platelets.[6] In two published series of transfused PPH patients, the portions of patients who received fresh frozen plasma (FFP) (27%[7] and 28%[8]), cryoprecipitate (7%[7] and 8%[8]), and platelets (16%[7] and 5%[8]) were lower, suggesting that accreta patients may have a higher baseline need for procoagulant blood component therapy. There are almost no specific data on the portion of transfused accreta patients who received other hemostatic agents such as tranexamic acid (TXA), fibrinogen concentrate, or recombinant factor VIIa (rFVIIa), but guidance on use of these products is available from studies on PPH. This chapter reviews blood management strategies; discusses patient blood management as it applies to individual patients with accreta; reviews blood products and their use; reviews hemostatic agents and their use in patients with accreta; and highlights new therapies and how they might be utilized in the future.

Blood Product Administration Strategies

Placenta accreta increases the potential for obstetric bleeding (bleeding originating from the blood vessels within the postpartum uterus), surgical bleeding (bleeding due to incisions, lacerations, or ruptured vessels), and coagulopathic bleeding (bleeding due to the loss or consumption of clotting factors and/or platelets) most frequently due to massive hemorrhage associated with either of the preceding. The goals in the management of massive hemorrhage are control of obstetrical and surgical bleeding (discussed elsewhere in this book); maintenance of perfusion and oxygenation by restoration of blood volume and hemoglobin (Hb)[9]; and judicious use of blood component therapy to correct coagulopathy.[9]

Adequacy of the Blood Bank and Transfusion Medicine Support

Maintenance of perfusion/oxygenation and correction of coagulopathy requires adequate support from the blood bank. The American College of Obstetrics and Gynecology (ACOG) Practice Bulletin on Placenta Accreta (2012) recommends that the blood bank be placed on alert for a potential massive hemorrhage.[10] This presumes that the blood bank has sufficient capacity—an important prerequisite in the care of the patient with accreta. Besides meeting newly developed criteria for a subspecialty care center or regional perinatal health care center,[11] a center should have an obstetric massive transfusion protocol and adequate inventory in the blood bank. To illustrate the importance of this point: in 2006, a Japanese obstetrician was arrested and charged with manslaughter in the death of a patient with accreta who died in 2004 as a consequence of massive hemorrhage after the hospital blood bank was exhausted.[12] A review of the case reveals that 2 hours after the start of the cesarean (which was after the fourth round of blood products, but prior to hysterectomy), the team was still awaiting the arrival of additional blood products.[12] Although the obstetrician was ultimately judged not guilty in 2008,[12] police had alleged that the obstetrician, "knew [the patient] was suffering from an adherent placenta and that the procedure could lead to considerable blood loss, yet failed to transfer the patient to a hospital with better facilities," (specifically those with an adequately stocked blood bank).[13] A recently published expert review states that one of the most important features of a center of excellence for patients with accreta is, "a state-of-the art, well-stocked blood bank that functions at full capacity 24 hours a day, 7 days a week," with "a well-established massive transfusion protocol."[14] The authors also cite an expanded role for the transfusion medicine specialist, who may need to assume management of blood product administration and even monitor the consequent electrolyte changes that accompany massive transfusion.

Massive Transfusion Protocols

The ACOG Practice Bulletin on Placenta Accreta (2012) also recommends that institutionally established massive transfusion protocols be followed. The National Partnership for Maternal Safety in the United States, which included representatives from the American Association of Blood Banks, ACOG, and the California Maternal Quality Care Collaborative (CMQCC), developed a consensus "bundle" for obstetric hemorrhage. The "bundle" is not a new guideline, but a package of existing guidelines/recommendations organized into four sections: Readiness; Recognition and Prevention; Response; and Reporting and Systems Learning. With respect to Readiness, the bundle recommends that every unit has: (1) a hemorrhage cart, (2) immediate access to medications, (3) a response team, (4) massive and emergency-release transfusion protocols (uncrossmatched, type-O negative RBCs), and (5) education and drills on the protocols.[15] The CMQCC emphasizes massive transfusion protocols that rapidly deliver blood products once activated.[16]

Obstetric massive hemorrhage protocols should have clear criteria for activation. Early recognition of excessive blood loss is critical. Vital sign changes may provide indications of excessive blood loss, with changes of heart rate, respiration, or blood pressure serving as a trigger, but it is important to remember that many obstetric patients (often young healthy women) will experience hypotension only after significant blood loss (1,500 mL or more). Visual estimates of blood loss have historically been employed in obstetrics, but they frequently underestimate actual blood loss, especially at larger volumes.[17] Quantitative assessments are preferred. Two quantitative assessment methods recommended by the CMQCC are: (1) weight of blood-soaked materials (i.e., pads, sponges) and (2) volume of blood captured in under-buttock graduated cylinder drapes.[15]

After observational studies of blood replacement in trauma suggested a 1:1 ratio of RBCs to plasma was associated with improved hemostasis and/or survival, this ratio was adopted in obstetric massive transfusion protocols. While there are no studies in obstetric patients, a recent randomized trial among patients with severe trauma and major bleeding found that early administration of plasma, platelets, and RBCs in a 1:1:1 ratio compared with a 1:1:2 ratio did not result in significant mortality differences at 24 hours or 30 days, but more patients in the 1:1:1 group achieved hemostasis and fewer died of exsanguination within the first 24 hours. There was an increased use of plasma and platelets in the 1:1:1 group, but no differences in adverse events between groups were identified.[18] Pregnant patients have a different coagulation profile at baseline compared to nonpregnant patients, which raises the question as to whether the results of trauma studies can be applied to obstetric patients, but in the absence of studies in obstetric patients, results from trauma studies are the best evidence available. Obstetric massive transfusion protocols that have incorporated higher RBC-to-plasma ratios between 1:1 and 2:1 have been successful in controlling hemorrhage and reducing blood product utilization.[19] The National Partnership for Maternal Safety consensus bundle for obstetric hemorrhage supports an RBC-to-plasma ratio between 1:1 and 2:1 for the total transfused units as well as the administration of a dose of apheresis platelets for approximately every six to eight units of RBCs; early coagulation testing and serial laboratory monitoring and, in some instances, point-of-care technologies to assess the maternal coagulation profile and guide ongoing correction; and the monitoring of fibrinogen levels and replacement with cryoprecipitate as needed.[15]

The Society for Advancement of Blood Management has provided guidelines for massive hemorrhage protocols on its website (https://www.sabm.org/sites/default/files/SABM_Admin-Standards3rdEdition .pdf).[20] These guidelines emphasize the multimodal approach to hemorrhage management and delineate elements which should be incorporated into protocols, including obstetric hemorrhage protocols (Table 10.1). While transfusion is a key element in these protocols, planning is also recommended for other elements such as laboratory testing and interpretation, metabolic complications of massive transfusion, and use of adjuvant pharmacotherapy such as antifibrinolytics and factor concentrates.

TABLE 10.1

Society for the Advancement of Blood Management (SABM) Selected Recommendations for Elements in Massive Hemorrhage Protocols (MHPs)

SABM Guideline	Obstetric-Specific Recommendations
10.1: There are defined criteria for starting and stopping the MHP	
10.3: Responsibility for management of coagulopathy is defined (among various disciplines)	Roles of other disciplines (anesthesiology, hematology, transfusion medicine) are defined
10.5: MHP includes guidelines for management of acidosis, hypocalcemia, and hypothermia	
10.6: MHP includes guidelines for blood component transfusion and factor concentrates	Refer to the California Maternal Quality Care Collaborative (CMQCC) recommendations
10.7: Laboratory testing is used to monitor for acidosis, hypocalcemia, and coagulation	Testing should be able to rapidly identify hypofibrinogenemia
10.8 Laboratory results are available quickly enough to allow for goal-directed transfusion	
10.10: There is multidisciplinary review of complex cases involving massive transfusion	Refer to National Partnership for Maternal Safety case review forms for severe maternal morbidity: http://www.safehealthcareforeverywoman.org/national-partnership.php

Source: Society for the Advancement of Blood Management I. *SABM Administrated and Clinical Standards for Patient Blood Management Programs.* 3rd Ed. Richmond, VA: Society for the Advancement of Blood Management; 2014.

Laboratory Monitoring

In accreta patients, a baseline coagulation laboratory assessment should be obtained at time of hemorrhage recognition to include platelet count, prothrombin time (PT), partial thromboplastin time (PTT), and fibrinogen levels. Reassessment should be performed if and when hemorrhage is recognized and repeated frequently (every 30–45 minutes) until the hemorrhage is controlled.[16,21] To ensure timely results for goal-directed therapy, standard coagulation testing can be optimized for improved turnaround times. Chandler and colleagues developed an emergency hemostasis panel (EHP) consisting of an Hb, platelet count, PT/INR, and fibrinogen level with a turnaround time of 14 ± 3 minutes, which significantly improved on the pre-EHP turnaround time of 35 ± 37 minutes.[22]

Hypofibrinogenemia has gained significant attention as an important predictor of severe PPH. Charbit and colleagues assessed coagulation laboratory values at the time of second-line uterotonic administration in 128 patients experiencing PPH. The only laboratory value which predicted progression to severe PPH, as defined by (1) transfusion of four or more packed RBC (pRBC) units, (2) Hb decrease of >4 g/dL, (3) procedural intervention, or (4) death, was a fibrinogen level <200 mg/dL.[23] A subanalysis of the PITHAGORE trial similarly identified fibrinogen levels <2 g/L as predictive of severe PPH.[24] In light of these data, rapid identification of hypofibrinogenemia is strongly recommended for patients experiencing obstetric hemorrhage.

Viscoelastic coagulation testing such as thromboelastography (TEG) or rotational thromboelastometry (ROTEM) can be employed for rapid hemostasis assessment;[25] see Figure 10.1. Similar to Clauss fibrinogen levels, detection of hyperfibrinogenemia by ROTEM in the setting of PPH has recently been shown to predict severe PPH.[26] A systematic review of nine randomized trials examining viscoelastic testing in hemorrhage, while not finding evidence of reduced patient morbidity or mortality, did find an association with reduced bleeding or transfusion.[27]

Furthermore, viscoelastic clot-based tests such as TEG and ROTEM are the only laboratory tests which can rapidly identify hyperfibrinolysis. Until data are available from large trials designed to evaluate safety and efficacy of empiric antifibrinolytic therapy in obstetric hemorrhage, laboratory testing can direct antifibrinolytic use for those patients with identified hyperfibrinolysis.

Anesthesia Management

Anticipating the potential for hemorrhage, and the corresponding requirement for fluid resuscitation and transfusion, is a core requirement of the successful anesthetic management of the patient with accreta.[28] In order for resuscitation and transfusion to be successful, the anesthesia team should be fully apprised of the

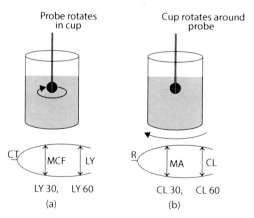

FIGURE 10.1 Viscoelastic coagulation: (a) rotational thromboelastometry (ROTEM) versus (b) thromboelastography (TEG). Clotting time (CT) (in minutes) reflects clotting factor activity; maximum strength (in millimeters) reflects platelets and fibrinogen; and % lysis (at a fixed time, e.g., 30 or 60 minutes) reflects fibrinolysis. (a) CT: maximum clot firmness (MCF), a measure of maximum strength; LY 30 = % clot lysis at 30 minutes; LY 60 = % clot lysis at 60 minutes. (b) Reaction time (R), a measure of clotting time, maximum amplitude (MA), a measure of maximum strength; CL 30 = % clot lysis at 30 minutes; CL 60 = % clot lysis at 60 minutes.

patient's condition well in advance of delivery, have the opportunity to meet with the patient in advance and have the opportunity to prepare the patient and the environment. Anesthesia considerations include large-bore venous access,[29] high-flow rate infusion and suction devices,[29] hemodynamic monitoring capabilities,[29] warming devices for fluids,[29] and, possibly, setup for cell salvage.[30] Communication among team members is essential during preparation for delivery and in monitoring ongoing blood loss during delivery.[28]

Coagulation factors function optimally at normal body temperature. Evidence suggests that hypothermia contributes to coagulopathy.[31,32] In terms of morbidity, the impact of hypothermia on coagulation is synergistic with that of acidosis.[32] To prevent hypothermia, the anesthesia team may use warming devices for fluids, may use forced air warming, and may increase the ambient temperature to maintain the patient's temperature between 36°C and 37.5°C.

Patient Blood Management

Patient blood management is an evidence-based, multidisciplinary approach to optimizing the care of patients who might need transfusion.[33] Patient blood management encompasses all aspects of patient evaluation and clinical management surrounding the transfusion decision-making process, including measures to avoid or minimize transfusion such as anemia management, cell salvage, and the use of hemostatic medication to reduce bleeding.[34]

Preoperative Autologous Donation

Preoperative autologous donation was primarily introduced to help eliminate infectious disease transmission at the time of transfusion,[35] but it is generally no longer recommended in obstetrics.[36] Autologous units as a percentage of all units collected peaked in 1992 at 8.5%, but as the real and perceived risk of infectious disease transmission has declined, collection of autologous units has declined as well to less than 0.2% of total units collected.[35] Currently, the risk of infection per unit of RBCs is approximately 1/1,470,000 for HIV, 1/1,150,000 for hepatitis C virus (HCV), and 1/765,000–1,010,000 for hepatitis B virus (HBV).[35] At present, the greatest risks in transfusion are noninfectious, such as transfusion-related acute lung injury (TRALI), transfusion-associated circulatory overload (TACO), or mistransfusion (the wrong blood transfused into the wrong patient)[37]; these risks are not obviated by autologous donation. Importantly, postdonation Hb levels may not return to baseline before delivery and donation may exacerbate anemia.[35] Additional theoretical risks of autologous donation in pregnancy include hypovolemia during the collection process and a decrease in maternal iron stores, both of which could potentially affect the fetus. Furthermore, autologous donation may not decrease the need for allogeneic transfusion.[36]

Anemia Management

Preoperative anemia management has been shown to reduce perioperative transfusion requirements.[38] In patients with accreta, an ideal preoperative Hb level has not been established, but anemia should be avoided. In pregnancy, anemia has been defined as an Hb <11.0 g/dL in the first trimester, <10.5 g/dL in the second and third trimesters, and <10.0 g/dL in the postpartum period.[39] In patients with accreta, iron deficiency anemia should be identified, and treated early and effectively. Women with iron deficiency anemia should receive 100–200 mg elemental iron daily.[39] There have been several randomized-controlled trials of oral versus intravenous iron in pregnant women.[40–46] Although both are effective in raising Hb levels, a 2 g/dL increase is more likely to be achieved within 4 weeks of starting therapy by intravenous than oral iron. For patients with iron deficiency anemia who cannot tolerate or fail to respond to oral iron, intravenous iron should be started as early as the second trimester.

The most serious risk of intravenous iron therapy is anaphylaxis and the risk differs by formulation. A recent retrospective study of Medicare patients receiving a first iron infusion found that the risk of anaphylaxis was 68 per 100,000 for iron dextran versus 24 per 100,000 for nondextran products (iron sucrose, gluconate, and ferumoxytol). When compared with iron sucrose, the adjusted odds ratio of anaphylaxis for iron dextran was 3.6 (95% CI, 2.4–5.4); for iron gluconate, 2.0 (95% CI 1.2, 3.5); and for ferumoxytol, 2.2 (95% CI, 1.1–4.3).[47]

Cell Salvage

Intraoperative cell salvage is another strategy to decrease the need for allogeneic blood transfusion. Historically, cell salvage has been avoided in obstetric patients because of the potential risk of amniotic fluid embolism or the risk of maternal alloimmunization to fetal RBC antigens. However, with advances in cell salvage technology, the risks in obstetric patients appear to be comparable to the risks in other patients. In obstetric patients, modifications are commonly made to the process, including (1) use of a separate suction source to waste blood and amniotic fluid collected before the delivery of the placenta and (2) addition of a leukocyte depletion filter to the circuit to reduce levels of contaminants prior to transfusion of autologous cell-salvaged blood. Fetal antigens remain, and in RhD negative patients, Rh immune globulin (RhIg) is required after a Kleihauer–Betke test is used to quantify the exposure and calculate the dose. In obstetric patients who received salvage blood, no definite cases of amniotic fluid embolism have been reported and no serious complications were reported in seven peer-reviewed studies of approximately 300 subjects.[30]

Blood Products

Red Blood Cells

RBCs contain Hb and transport oxygen, carbon dioxide, and nitric oxide. pRBCs are prepared for transfusion by centrifugation of whole blood or by apheresis with removal of plasma. RBCs are anticoagulated with citrate and may have one or more preservative solutions added to prolong shelf life. Depending on the anticoagulant–preservative system used, the resulting RBCs have a hematocrit of 55%–65% to 65%–80% and a usual volume of 300–400 mL.[48] Ideally, serologic compatibility should be established before RBCs are transfused. ABO-group specific pRBC units can be issued within 10–15 minutes; fully crossmatched units for patients with RBC alloantibodies may take significantly longer (45 minutes or more). In an emergency, uncrossmatched type O-negative RBCs may be issued if the delay in compatibility testing could be life-threatening for the patient. Each unit has the capacity to increase the Hb concentration of the average adult by 1 g/dL and the hematocrit by 3%.[49] RBCs are recommended in order to maintain a hematocrit >24%[15] or an Hb of >8 g/dL,[50] and between 7.0 and 10 g/dL during active bleeding.[51]

Plasma Components

Patients undergoing massive transfusion who have clinically significant coagulation deficiencies require plasma transfusion. Important elements in plasma include albumin, coagulation factors, fibrinolytic proteins, immunoglobulins, and anticoagulant proteins. Plasma is derived from the centrifugation of whole blood or by apheresis. Once plasma is collected, it typically is frozen for up to a year and subsequently thawed. Similar to RBCs, plasma units are anticoagulated with citrate. On average, units contain 200–250 mL, but apheresis-derived units may contain as much as 400–600 mL.[48] FFP is prepared from a whole blood or apheresis collection and frozen at ≤–18°C within 8 hours of collection. In contrast, plasma frozen within 24 hours after phlebotomy (FP24) is frozen within 24 hours of collection.[48] Both FFP and FP24 should be transfused immediately after thawing or stored at 1°C–6°C for no more than 24 hours.[48] After 24 hours, these products may be relabeled as "thawed plasma" for use within 5 days following the initial thaw. While levels of labile factors such as factor V, factor VIII, and protein C are somewhat reduced in FP24 and thawed plasma as compared to FFP,[48] these products are considered of roughly equal hemostatic potency for hemorrhage management in adults. Thawed plasma not only reduces wastage of plasma but also provides rapidly available plasma for massive hemorrhage. Plasma is almost always issued as ABO-compatible to the patient, with group AB plasma issued as the most common form of universally compatible emergency released plasma. In some centers, small amounts of group A plasma may be released as an alternative to group AB plasma due to the scarcity of AB blood type.[52] The target of therapy is an activated partial thromboplastin time (aPTT) <1.5 × normal and a PT <1.5 × normal.[53]

Cryoprecipitate

Cryoprecipitate serves as a source of fibrinogen, factor VIII, factor XIII, and von Willebrand factor (VWF). Cryoprecipitate is used in the management of hemorrhage associated with fibrinogen deficiency and the treatment of single-factor deficiencies when specific factor concentrates are not available. Cryoprecipitate is prepared by thawing whole blood-derived FFP between 1°C and 6°C and recovering the precipitate. In the United States, each unit of cryoprecipitate should contain ≥80 IU factor VIII and ≥150 mg of fibrinogen in approximately 5–20 mL of plasma.[48] Cryoprecipitate may be transfused as individual units or pooled. The label indicates if several units have been pooled together and gives the volume of the pool.[48] If used, 0.9% sodium chloride, the preferred diluent, may be listed separately.[48] When used to correct hypofibrinogenemia, cryoprecipitate may be dosed by formula or empirically. An individual unit can increase fibrinogen levels by up to 10 mg/dL and a five-unit cryoprecipitate pool can increase fibrinogen levels by 25–50 mg/dL,[54] but response can vary widely due to the heterogeneous composition of cryoprecipitate, the rate of consumption, degree of fibrinogen recovery, and half-life. That half-life is approximately 4 days in the absence of increased consumption (e.g., bleeding or disseminated intravascular coagulation). The patient's pretransfusion and posttransfusion fibrinogen levels should be determined to assess the adequacy of the cryoprecipitate dose. Cryoprecipitate is acellular and compatibility testing is unnecessary, but ABO-compatible units are preferred. RhD type need not be considered when using this component.[49] The target of therapy is a PT <1.5 × normal and, based on new evidence discussed later, a fibrinogen of ≥200 mg/dL.[53]

Platelets

Platelet transfusions may be given to patients with thrombocytopenia, dysfunctional platelet disorders (congenital, metabolic, or medication-induced), or active platelet-related bleeding, and to patients at serious risk of bleeding (i.e., prophylactic use). Platelets are prepared by apheresis or derived from whole blood, then suspended in an appropriate volume of the original plasma, which contains near-normal levels of stable coagulation factors. Apheresis platelets may be stored in either citrated plasma or an additive solution. A unit of apheresis platelets contains $\geq 3.0 \times 10^{11}$ platelets in 100–500 mL of plasma or plasma plus additive solution, and is the therapeutic equivalent of four to six units of whole blood-derived platelets.[48] A unit of whole blood-derived platelets contains $\geq 5.5 \times 10^{10}$ platelets suspended in 40–70 mL of plasma.[48] Platelets are stored at room temperature with a 5-day shelf life.[48] Compatibility testing is not necessary in routine platelet transfusion. Except in unusual circumstances, the donor plasma should be ABO compatible with the recipient's RBCs to prevent hemolysis when large volumes are to be transfused.[48] One unit of whole blood-derived platelets would be expected to increase the platelet count of a 70-kg adult by 5,000–10,000/μL,[49] with one apheresis platelet transfusion expected to give a posttransfusion increment of 30,000–50,000/μL. During uncontrolled hemorrhage, the target platelet count should be at least 50,000/μL.[53] While platelets do not bear RhD antigens, trace amounts of RBCs in this product necessitate providing RhD-negative platelets to RhD-negative women. Should RhD-negative platelets not be available, a dose of RhIg can be provided to prevent alloimmunization.[55]

Blood product replacement recommendations are summarized in Table 10.2, with target hematologic target values summarized in Table 10.3. An example of a single institution's (Duke University Medical Center's) algorithm is provided in Table 10.4.

Hemostatic Agents

Antifibrinolytic Therapy

Antifibrinolytic therapy has been used infrequently in the United States for the prevention or management of PPH, but favorable data are accumulating that may change practice. After TXA was shown in two randomized trials of uncertain quality to decrease postpartum blood loss after vaginal birth and after cesarean delivery,[56] two subsequent randomized-controlled trials have been published and one is underway. Xu et al.[57] compared intravenous TXA (10 mg/kg) versus placebo to prevent blood loss at the time of cesarean delivery in 174 primipara. Blood loss up to 2 hours postpartum was significantly lower in

TABLE 10.2

Blood Product Replacement

Product	Volume	Contents	Effect
Packed red blood cells (pRBCs)	300–400 mL	RBCs, residual leukocytes, and plasma	Increases hematocrit by 3%; hemoglobin by 1 g/dL
Plasma	200–250 mL (apheresis units may contain 400–600 mL)	All soluble clotting factors, anticoagulant proteins, and fibrinogen	Can increase fibrinogen up to 10 mg/dL
Cryoprecipitate	~40 mL	Fibrinogen, factors VIII and XIII, and von Willebrand factor	Widely variable
Platelets—whole blood	40–70 mL	Platelets, RBCs, white blood cells, and plasma	Increases platelet count by 5,000–10,000/µL
Platelets—apheresis	100–500 mL	Platelets, RBCs, white blood cells, and plasma	Increases platelet count by 30,000–50,000/µL

Sources: American Association of Blood Banks (AABB) et al., *Circular of Information for the Use of Human Blood and Blood Components*, 2013; Vassallo R et al., *A Compendium of Transfusion Practice Guidelines*, American Red Cross, Washington, DC, 2013.

TABLE 10.3

Recommended Hematologic Targets Following Transfusion

Parameter	Target
Hematocrit	>24%
Hemoglobin	>8 g/dL (between 7.0 and 10 g/dL during active bleeding)
Prothrombin time (PT)	<1.5 × normal
Activate partial thromboplastin time (aPTT)	<1.5 × normal
Platelet count	>50,000/µL
Fibrinogen	>200 g/dL

TABLE 10.4

Duke University Medical Center Algorithm for Transfusion and Laboratory Evaluation in Obstetric Hemorrhage

Evaluate:

Draw the following labs every 30 minutes:
- Hematocrit
- Hemoglobin
- Platelet count
- PT/INR[a]
- aPTT
- Fibrinogen

Replace:

Parameter
- Platelet count <50,000/µL
- INR >1.5
- Fibrinogen <150 mg/dL

Transfuse
- 1 apheresis platelet
- 2–4 units plasma
- 1 pool cryoprecipitate

Manage massive hemorrhage:

1. Transfuse RBCs and plasma in 1:1 ratio—alternate RBCs and FFP units.
2. After 6 RBCs and 6 plasma units, transfuse 1 apheresis platelet.
3. After an additional 6 RBCs and 6 plasma units, transfuse 1 pool cryoprecipitate.

[a]INR, International normalized ratio

the TXA group than in the control group. Ducloy-Bouthors[58] published the results of intravenous TXA (loading dose 4 g over 1 hour, then an infusion of 1 g/hour over 6 hours) versus no therapy for secondary prevention of PPH in 144 women with an estimated blood loss at delivery of >800 mL following vaginal delivery. Blood loss 6 hours later was significantly lower in the TXA group than in the control group. There were two catheter-related thromboses in the TXA group which was not a statistically significant difference, but the study was not powered to detect a difference in thromboses.[58] A very large, international multicenter trial, the World Maternal Antifibrinolytic (WOMAN) Trial, has recently completed recruiting subjects. Inclusion criteria were an estimated blood loss ≥500 mL after vaginal delivery or ≥1,000 mL after cesarean delivery. Subjects were randomized to 1–2 g intravenous TXA versus saline.[59] Results should be available later this year. TXA may be a useful adjunct in the management of obstetric hemorrhage and has now been included in some obstetric massive transfusion protocols. Table 10.5 reviews guidelines from obstetric, anesthesia, and hematology societies within the last 5 years regarding use of TXA in obstetric hemorrhage.[53,60,61]

Recombinant Factor VIIa

rFVIIa is indicated for the prevention or treatment of bleeding in hemophilia patients with inhibitors, but has been used in the management of severe PPH, primarily in cases unresponsive to blood component therapy. The combination of FVIIa with tissue factor initiates the clotting cascade; see Figure 10.2. In a survey of off-label use of rFVIIa, more than 70% was used in cardiac surgery, 7% in trauma, and less than 1% in obstetrics.[62] The largest reported series of the off-label use of rFVIIa in obstetrics is from the Australian and New Zealand Haemostasis Registry.[63] The investigators recorded all off-label use of rFVIIa for treatment of acute PPH in 105 cases; accreta accounted for 16% of the patients. The majority (78%) received a single dose (median dose = 92 mcg/kg) with a positive response in 76% (64% after a single dose). Two women developed venous thromboembolism. The Northern Europe Factor 7a in Obstetric Hemorrhage Study reported rFVIIa use in 92 women with

TABLE 10.5

Tranexamic Acid (TXA) Guideline Recommendations (within Last 5 Years)

Organization/Group	Recommendation
European Society of Anaesthesia (2013)[60]	Administer TXA to reduce blood loss, bleeding duration, and transfusion requirements (Grade 1B)
WHO (2012)[61]	For refractory atonic and trauma-related bleeding (weak recommendation, moderate evidence)
ISTH (2015)[53]	Suggest that women with ongoing postpartum hemorrhage (PPH) be considered to receive 1 g TXA

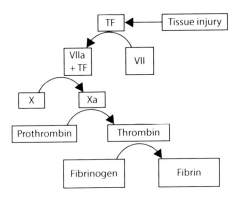

FIGURE 10.2 Initiation of the clotting cascade showing the role of factor VIIa and fibrinogen.

obstetric hemorrhage. The majority (81%) received a single dose. The most common was 90 mcg/kg with a positive response of 86% (80% after a single dose).[64] Four women developed venous thromboembolism. If rFVIIa has a role in the management of accreta, it is in achieving hemostasis after hysterectomy when conventional hemostatic management has failed. When effective, an improvement in bleeding should be seen within 10–15 minutes after administration of the drug. If the first dose is judged to be ineffective, a second dose may be tried, but further doses are not recommended. When used, the Australia and New Zealand guidelines suggest dosing at 90 mcg/kg. Whether lower doses are effective in obstetrics is unknown. Because of the recognized thromboembolic risk, the European Society of Anesthesia recommended rFVIIa be considered only as a last-line therapy for obstetric hemorrhage.[60]

Clinicians who are considering use of rFVIIa in uncontrolled PPH should optimize the patient's hemostatic potential, with correction of hypofibrinogenemia, clotting factor deficiency, and thrombocytopenia prior to administration. Failure to optimize fibrinogen can result in a lack of response to rFVIIa.[65] In addition, the patient ideally should have a pH of 7.2 or greater, as rFVIIa activity significantly decreases in acidosis.[66]

Fibrinogen Concentrate

Historically, standard practice was to replace fibrinogen to maintain a level of ≥100 mg/dL as this level is thought to be sufficient to promote normal hemostasis,[67] but with identification of fibrinogen <200 mg/dL as a biomarker for progression to severe PPH,[23,24] higher fibrinogen levels may be required for hemostasis at the time of delivery. Cryoprecipitate is preferred to plasma to correct low fibrinogen levels; however, concerns regarding the risk of pathogen transmission have led to the substitution or partial substitution of virally inactivated fibrinogen concentrates, particularly in Europe. Multiple case reports and small series of its use in the management of obstetrical hemorrhage have been published.[68–71] Doses ranging from 2 to 4 g were given alone or in combination with plasma or cryoprecipitate with hemorrhage described as "improved" and coagulopathy described as "resolved." A randomized-controlled trial conducted at four hospitals in Denmark compared the preemptive administration of fibrinogen concentrate (2 g intravenously) versus saline in patients with normal fibrinogen levels who had estimated blood loss of ≥500 mL after vaginal delivery or ≥1,000 mL after cesarean delivery. There was no difference in the rate of transfusion between the two groups (nor were there any thromboembolic events in either group).[72] Whether fibrinogen concentrate is useful (1) in patients who are hypofibrinogenemic or (2) at a higher dose, is unknown. Table 10.6 summarizes recommendations from obstetric, anesthesia, and hematology societies regarding fibrinogen repletion goals in obstetric hemorrhage.[16,53,60]

Prothrombin Complex Concentrates

Prothrombin complex concentrates (PCCs) are virally inactivated concentrates of factors II, VII, IX, and X. PCCs with low amounts of FVII (three-factor PCCs) were originally used as a treatment for hemophilia B. PCCs containing sufficient FVII levels (four-factor PCCs) are now used for acute reversal of vitamin K antagonists.[73] A potential advantage of PCCs over plasma is the lower volume required to restore clotting

TABLE 10.6

Fibrinogen (Fgn) Replacement Guideline Recommendations (within Last 5 Years)

Organization/Group	Recommendation
European Society of Anaesthesia (2013)[60]	• Fgn <2 g/L may indicate increased risk for PPH (Grade 2C) • Fgn <1.5–2.0 g/L deficit should be triggers for Fgn substitution (Grade 1C)
California Maternal Quality Care Collaborative (2015)[16]	• Initial order for cryoprecipitate when Fgn <100 mg/dL or if patient has severe abruption or amniotic fluid embolism • Maintain Fgn >100–125 mg/dL
ISTH (2015)[4]	• Suggest maintaining Fgn >2 g/L with cryoprecipitate or fibrinogen concentrates

factors and their pathogen inactivation.[73] A disadvantage is that formulations differ and some contain heparin.[74] There are anecdotal reports of the use of PCCs in massive hemorrhage,[73] but no studies have demonstrated their efficacy and, as of yet, there are no reports of their use in obstetric hemorrhage.

New Developments in Blood Component Pathogen Reduction

Two systems for blood component pathogen reduction have been approved for use within the United States. Although the US blood supply is safer than ever before, some bacteria, viruses, prions, and parasites can still be transmitted. The Intercept System (Cerus, Concord, CA) uses a psoralen which binds pathogen nucleic acid and is activated by ultraviolet A (UVA) light, preventing pathogen replication. While pathogens (bacteria, viruses, and parasites) require replication of nucleic acids in order to transmit infection, platelets, plasma, and RBCs do not require functional DNA or RNA for their survival or therapeutic efficacy. Currently, the system is approved in the United States for pathogen reduction in both plasma and platelets, with ongoing development for use in pRBCs. Octaplas® (Octapharma, Hoboken, NJ) is another pathogen-reduced plasma. It is produced in pools from 630 to 1,520 donors which undergo filtration and solvent-detergent reagent treatment to inactivate lipid-enveloped viruses, and affinity column filtration to reduce prion protein.[49] Units are supplied in ABO-specific 200-mL volumes.[49]

Summary

Patients with placenta accreta often require large-volume transfusion at time of delivery. It is, therefore, critical that these patients be delivered at centers with well-equipped transfusion services, adequate blood component inventories, and massive transfusion protocols. Empiric transfusion of blood components may be required, with available evidence supporting RBCs to plasma transfusion ratios of 1:1 to 2:1, with transfusion of platelets following every six to eight RBC units. Frequent laboratory monitoring using standard coagulation tests (including viscoelastic testing) is recommended for rapid identification of coagulopathy and directing goal-directed transfusion therapy while hemorrhage is uncontrolled. Patient blood management strategies, including antepartum anemia treatment and cell salvage, are useful in reducing allogeneic transfusion. While hemostatic agents—including antifibrinolytic agents, rFVIIa, fibrinogen concentrates, and PCCs—have limited data supporting their widespread use at this time, current and future clinical trials will likely demonstrate an important role for adjuvant pharmacotherapy in blood management for patients with accreta.

Conflict of Interest

Andra James has received honoraria and served on Advisory Committees for CSL Behring, Grifols, and Baxalta. Evelyn Lockhart has received honoraria from CSL Behring, TEM Systems Inc., and Octapharma and served on an Advisory Committee for CSL Behring, Bayer, Cerus, Octapharma, and TEM Systems Inc.

REFERENCES

1. Eller AG, Porter TF, Soisson P, Silver RM. Optimal management strategies for placenta accreta. *BJOG.* 2009;116:648–654.
2. Sentilhes L, Ambroselli C, Kayem G, et al. Maternal outcome after conservative treatment of placenta accreta. *Obstet Gynecol.* 2010;115:526–534.
3. Eller AG, Bennett MA, Sharshiner M, et al. Maternal morbidity in cases of placenta accreta managed by a multidisciplinary care team compared with standard obstetric care. *Obstet Gynecol.* 2011;117:331–337.

4. Mehrabadi A, Hutcheon JA, Liu S, et al. Contribution of placenta accreta to the incidence of postpartum hemorrhage and severe postpartum hemorrhage. *Obstet Gynecol.* 2015;125:814–821.

5. Shamshirsaz AA, Fox KA, Salmanian B, et al. Maternal morbidity in patients with morbidly adherent placenta treated with and without a standardized multidisciplinary approach. *Am J Obstet Gynecol.* 2015;212:218 e211–219.

6. Stotler B, Padmanabhan A, Devine P, Wright J, Spitalnik SL, Schwartz J. Transfusion requirements in obstetric patients with placenta accreta. *Transfusion.* 2011;51:2627–2633.

7. Butwick AJ, Aleshi P, Fontaine M, Riley ET, Goodnough LT. Retrospective analysis of transfusion outcomes in pregnant patients at a tertiary obstetric center. *Int J Obstet Anesth.* 2009;18:302–308.

8. James AH, Paglia MJ, Gernsheimer T, Grotegut C, Thames B. Blood component therapy in postpartum hemorrhage. *Transfusion.* 2009;49:2430–2433.

9. Stainsby D, MacLennan S, Thomas D, Isaac J, Hamilton PJ. Guidelines on the management of massive blood loss. *Br J Haematol.* 2006;135:634–641.

10. Committee on Obstetric Practice. Committee opinion no. 529: Placenta accreta. *Obstet Gynecol.* 2012;120:207–211.

11. Menard MK, Kilpatrick S, Saade G, et al. Levels of maternal care. *Am J Obstet Gynecol.* 2015;212:259–271.

12. Higuchi, N. Should medical accidents be judged in criminal court? Case III: The case of Fukushima prefectural Ono Hospital—Chronology of Events. *Japan Med Assoc J.* 2012;55:128–137.

13. Doctor held over botched Caesarean. *The Japan Times*, February 19, 2006.

14. Silver RM, Fox KA, Barton JR, et al. Center of excellence for placenta accreta. *Am J Obstet Gynecol.* 2015;212:561–568.

15. Main EK, Goffman D, Scavone BM, et al. National partnership for maternal safety: Consensus bundle on obstetric hemorrhage. *Obstet Gynecol.* 2015;126:155–162.

16. Lyndon A, Lagrew D, Shields LE, Main E, Cape V. A California toolkit to transform maternity care. In: Obstetric Hemorrhage Task Force; California Maternal Quality Care Collaborative (CMQCC); Maternal Child and Adolescent Health Division; Centre for Family Health; California Department of Public Health, eds. *Improving Health Care Response to Obstetric Hemorrhage Version 2.0: A California Quality Improvement Toolkit.* Sacramento, CA: California Department of Public Health; 2015:1–179.

17. Lilley G, Burkett-St-Laurent D, Precious E, et al. Measurement of blood loss during postpartum haemorrhage. *Int J Obstet Anesth.* 2015;24:8–14.

18. Holcomb JB, Tilley BC, Baraniuk S, et al. Transfusion of plasma, platelets, and red blood cells in a 1:1:1 vs a 1:1:2 ratio and mortality in patients with severe trauma: The PROPPR randomized clinical trial. *JAMA.* 2015;313:471–482.

19. Shields LE, Smalarz K, Reffigee L, Mugg S, Burdumy TJ, Propst M. Comprehensive maternal hemorrhage protocols improve patient safety and reduce utilization of blood products. *Am J Obstet Gynecol.* 2011;205:368 e361–368.

20. Society for the Advancement of Blood Management I. *SABM Administrated and Clinical Standards for Patient Blood Management Programs.* 3rd Ed. Richmond, VA: Society for the Advancement of Blood Management; 2014.

21. Abdul-Kadir R, McLintock C, Ducloy AS, et al. Evaluation and management of postpartum hemorrhage: Consensus from an international expert panel. *Transfusion.* 2014;54:1756–1768.

22. Chandler WL, Ferrell C, Trimble S, Moody S. Development of a rapid emergency hemorrhage panel. *Transfusion.* 2010;50:2547–2552.

23. Charbit B, Mandelbrot L, Samain E, et al. The decrease of fibrinogen is an early predictor of the severity of postpartum hemorrhage. *J Thromb Haemost.* 2007;5:266–273.

24. Cortet M, Deneux-Tharaux C, Dupont C, et al. Association between fibrinogen level and severity of postpartum haemorrhage: Secondary analysis of a prospective trial. *Br J Anaesth.* 2012;108:984–989.

25. Ducloy-Bouthors AS, Susen S, Wong CA, Butwick A, Vallet B, Lockhart E. Medical advances in the treatment of postpartum hemorrhage. *Anesth Analg.* 2014;119:1140–1147.

26. Collins PW, Lilley G, Bruynseels D, et al. Fibrin-based clot formation as an early and rapid biomarker for progression of postpartum hemorrhage: A prospective study. *Blood.* 2014;124:1727–1736.

27. Afshari A, Wikkelso A, Brok J, Moller AM, Wetterslev J. Thrombelastography (TEG) or thromboelastometry (ROTEM) to monitor haemotherapy versus usual care in patients with massive transfusion. *Cochrane Database Syst Reviews.* 2011;(3): CD007871.

28. Dutton RP, Lee LA, Stephens LS, Posner KL, Davies JM, Domino KB. Massive hemorrhage: A report from the Anesthesia Closed Claims Project. *Anesthesiology.* 2014;121:450–458.
29. Belfort MA. Placenta accreta. *Am J Obstet Gynecol.* 2010;203:430–439.
30. Goucher H, Wong CA, Patel SK, Toledo P. Cell salvage in obstetrics. *Anesth Analg.* 2015;121:465–468.
31. Eddy VA, Morris JA Jr., Cullinane DC. Hypothermia, coagulopathy, and acidosis. *Surg Clin North Am.* 2000;80:845–854.
32. Dirkmann D, Hanke AA, Gorlinger K, Peters J. Hypothermia and acidosis synergistically impair coagulation in human whole blood. *Anesth Analg.* 2008;106:1627–1632.
33. Advancing Transfusion and Cellular Therapies Worldwide. Patient blood management. Available at: http://www.aabb.org/pbm/Pages/default.aspx?gclid=CjwKEAiAkvmzBRDQpozmt-uluCQSJACvCdll6DL9AmmJHLdf3GsOvZV4eWnKHHsejtgiFOESMzZEzBoCpfPw_wcB. Accessed on December 26, 2015.
34. Murphy MF, Goodnough LT. The scientific basis for patient blood management. *Transfus Clin Biol.* 2015;22:90–96.
35. Vassallo R, Goldman M, Germain M, Lozano M. Preoperative autologous blood donation: Waning indications in an era of improved blood safety. *Transfus Med Rev.* 2015;29:268–275.
36. Liumbruno GM, Liumbruno C, Rafanelli D. Autologous blood in obstetrics: Where are we going now? *Blood Transfus.* 2012;10:125–147.
37. American Association of Blood Banks. Decision making process for transfusion and transplantation safety policies: AABB statement before the Advisory Committee on Blood Safety and Availability 2009. Available at: http://www.aabb.org/advocacy/statements/Pages/statement050109.aspx. Accessed on December 26, 2015.
38. Guinn NR, Guercio JR, Hopkins TJ, et al. How do we develop and implement a preoperative anemia clinic designed to improve perioperative outcomes and reduce cost? *Transfusion.* 2015;56(2):297–303.
39. Pavord S, Myers B, Robinson S, Allard S, Strong J, Oppenheimer C. UK guidelines on the management of iron deficiency in pregnancy. *Br J Haematol.* 2012;156:588–600.
40. Shafi D, Purandare SV, Sathe AV. Iron deficiency anemia in pregnancy: Intravenous versus oral route. *J Obstet Gynaecol India.* 2012;62:317–321.
41. Kochhar PK, Kaundal A, Ghosh P. Intravenous iron sucrose versus oral iron in treatment of iron deficiency anemia in pregnancy: A randomized clinical trial. *J Obstet Gynaecol Res.* 2013;39:504–510.
42. Froessler B, Cocchiaro C, Saadat-Gilani K, Hodyl N, Dekker G. Intravenous iron sucrose versus oral iron ferrous sulfate for antenatal and postpartum iron deficiency anemia: A randomized trial. *J Matern Fetal Neonatal Med.* 2013;26:654–659.
43. Al-Momen AK, al-Meshari A, al-Nuaim L, et al. Intravenous iron sucrose complex in the treatment of iron deficiency anemia during pregnancy. *Eur J Obstet Gynecol Reprod Biol.* 1996;69:121–124.
44. Bayoumeu F, Subiran-Buisset C, Baka NE, Legagneur H, Monnier-Barbarino P, Laxenaire MC. Iron therapy in iron deficiency anemia in pregnancy: Intravenous route versus oral route. *Am J Obstet Gynecol.* 2002;186:518–522.
45. Shi Q, Leng W, Wazir R, et al. Intravenous iron sucrose versus oral iron in the treatment of pregnancy with iron deficiency anaemia: A systematic review. *Gynecol Obstet Invest.* 2015;80:170–178.
46. Al RA, Unlubilgin E, Kandemir O, Yalvac S, Cakir L, Haberal A. Intravenous versus oral iron for treatment of anemia in pregnancy: A randomized trial. *Obstet Gynecol.* 2005;106:1335–1340.
47. Wang C, Graham DJ, Kane RC, et al. Comparative risk of anaphylactic reactions associated with intravenous iron products. *JAMA.* 2015;314:2062–2068.
48. American Association of Blood Banks, American Red Cross, America's Blood Centers, and Armed Services Blood Program, Washington, D.C. *Circular of Information for the Use of Human Blood and Blood Components.* 2013:1–72. http://www.fda.gov/downloads/BiologicsBloodVaccines/GuidanceComplianceRegulatoryInformation/Guidances/Blood/UCM364587.pdf. Accessed on December 26, 2015.
49. Vassallo R, Bachowski G, Benjamin RJ, et al. In: Vassallo R, Ed. *A Compendium of Transfusion Practice Guidelines.* Washington, DC: American Red Cross; 2013. http://www.redcrossblood.org/sites/arc/files/59802_compendium_brochure_v_6_10_9_13.pdf.
50. Sentilhes L, Vayssiere C, Deneux-Tharaux C, et al. Postpartum hemorrhage: Guidelines for clinical practice from the French College of Gynaecologists and Obstetricians (CNGOF): In collaboration with the French Society of Anesthesiology and Intensive Care (SFAR). *Eur J Obstet Gynecol Reprod Biol.* 2016;198:12–21.

51. Bonnet MP, Deneux-Tharaux C, Dupont C, Rudigoz RC, Bouvier-Colle MH. Transfusion practices in postpartum hemorrhage: A population-based study. *Acta obstet Gynecol Scand.* 2013;92:404–413.

52. Cooling L. Going from A to B: The safety of incompatible group A plasma for emergency release in trauma and massive transfusion patients. *Transfusion.* 2014;54:1695–1697.

53. Collins P, Abdul-Kadir R, Thachil J. Management of coagulopathy associated with postpartum hemorrhage: Guidance from the SSC of the ISTH. *J Thromb Haemost.* 2016;14:205–210.

54. Callum JL, Karkouti K, Lin Y. Cryoprecipitate: The current state of knowledge. *Transfus Med Rev.* 2009;23:177–188.

55. Valsami S, Dimitroulis D, Gialeraki A, Chimonidou M, Politou M. Current trends in platelet transfusions practice: The role of ABO-RhD and human leukocyte antigen incompatibility. *Asian J Transfus Sci.* 2015;9:117–123.

56. Novikova N, Hofmeyr GJ. Tranexamic acid for preventing postpartum haemorrhage. *Cochrane Database Syst Rev.* 2010;(7):CD007872.

57. Xu J, Gao W, Ju Y. Tranexamic acid for the prevention of postpartum hemorrhage after cesarean section: A double-blind randomization trial. *Arch Gynecol Obstet.* 2013;287:463–468.

58. Ducloy-Bouthors AS, Jude B, Duhamel A, et al. High-dose tranexamic acid reduces blood loss in postpartum haemorrhage. *Crit Care.* 2011;15:R117.

59. World Maternal Antibrinolytic Trial (WOMAN). 2012. https://clinicaltrials.gov/ct2/show/NCT00872469. Accessed on December 15, 2015.

60. Kozek-Langenecker SA, Afshari A, Albaladejo P, et al. Management of severe perioperative bleeding: Guidelines from the European Society of Anaesthesiology. *Eur J Anaesthesiol.* 2013;30:270–382.

61. WHO. *WHO Recommendations for the Prevention and Treatment of Postpartum Haemorrhage.* Geneva: Department of Reproductive Health and Research, World Health Organization; 2012.

62. Andersen ND, Bhattacharya SD, Williams JB, et al. Intraoperative use of low-dose recombinant activated factor VII during thoracic aortic operations. *Ann Thorac Surg.* 2012;93:1921–1928; discussion 1928–1929.

63. Phillips LE, McLintock C, Pollock W, et al. Recombinant activated factor VII in obstetric hemorrhage: Experiences from the Australian and New Zealand Haemostasis Registry. *Anesth Analg.* 2009;109:1908–1915.

64. Alfirevic Z, Elbourne D, Pavord S, et al. Use of recombinant activated factor VII in primary postpartum hemorrhage: The Northern European registry 2000–2004. *Obstet Gynecol.* 2007;110:1270–1278.

65. Lewis NR, Brunker P, Lemire SJ, Kaufman RM. Failure of recombinant factor VIIa to correct the coagulopathy in a case of severe postpartum hemorrhage. *Transfusion.* 2009;49:689–695.

66. Meng ZH, Wolberg AS, Monroe DM, 3rd, Hoffman M. The effect of temperature and pH on the activity of factor VIIa: Implications for the efficacy of high-dose factor VIIa in hypothermic and acidotic patients. *J Trauma.* 2003;55:886–891.

67. Francois KE, Foley MR. Antepartum and postpartum hemorrhage. In: Gabbe S, Niebyl J, Simpson J, Eds. *Obstetrics: Normal and Problem Pregnancies*, 5th ed. Philadelphia, PA: Churchill Livingstone Elsevier; 2007:456–485.

68. Bell SF, Rayment R, Collins PW, Collis RE. The use of fibrinogen concentrate to correct hypofibrinogenaemia rapidly during obstetric haemorrhage. *Int J Obstet Anesth.* 2010;19:218–223.

69. Fenger-Eriksen C, Lindberg-Larsen M, Christensen AQ, Ingerslev J, Sorensen B. Fibrinogen concentrate substitution therapy in patients with massive haemorrhage and low plasma fibrinogen concentrations. *Br J Anaesth.* 2008;101:769–773.

70. Glover NJ, Collis RE, Collins P. Fibrinogen concentrate use during major obstetric haemorrhage. *Anaesthesia.* 2010;65:1229–1230.

71. Thorarinsdottir HR, Sigurbjornsson FT, Hreinsson K, Onundarson PT, Gudbjartsson T, Sigurdsson GH. Effects of fibrinogen concentrate administration during severe hemorrhage. *Acta Anaesthesiol Scand.* 2010;54:1077–1082.

72. Wikkelso AJ, Edwards HM, Afshari A, et al. Pre-emptive treatment with fibrinogen concentrate for postpartum haemorrhage: Randomized controlled trial. *Br J Anaesth.* 2015;114:623–633.

73. Tanaka KA, Szlam F. Treatment of massive bleeding with prothrombin complex concentrate: Argument for. *J Thromb Haemost.* 2010;8:2589–2591.

74. Godier A, Susen S, Samama CM. Treatment of massive bleeding with prothrombin complex concentrate: Argument against. *J Thromb Haemost.* 2010;8:2592–2595.

11

Anesthetic Considerations for Placenta Accreta

Erin Martin and Thomas Archer

CONTENTS

Introduction

The management of placenta accreta is complicated and requires the orchestration of numerous moving parts: multiple patients (mother and fetus), multiple locations (interventional radiology and operating room), multiple specialists (obstetricians, gynecologic oncologists, anesthesiologists, interventional radiologists, urologists, neonatologists, and nurses), and multiple procedures (endovascular interventions, ureteral stent placement, cesarean delivery, and gravid hysterectomy). Adding to this complexity, delivering a patient with placenta accreta is both a happy event resulting in the birth of a baby and a life-threatening event involving potentially torrential blood loss. In this context, anesthesiologists are placed in the middle of an interesting game of tug-of-war.

Optimal surgical exposure, hemodynamic stability, maternal airway protection, decreased neonatal drug exposure, early skin-to-skin contact between the mother and neonate, and postoperative pain control are all desirable goals but often are met with compromise when creating an anesthetic plan. Decisions regarding type of anesthesia, required monitoring, and invasive line placement should be made on a case-by-case basis depending on patient characteristics, extent of placental invasion, amount of expected hemorrhage, and practitioner preference.

Once a patient with placenta accreta is identified, scheduling an anesthesia consultation and multidisciplinary clinical care conference is paramount to ensuring a safe and successful delivery. Open communication and advanced planning among various members of the care team are essential to proper management. Additionally, these patients are best cared for in referral centers with appropriate breadth of experience and coverage.[1,2] This chapter represents an obstetrical anesthesiologist's perspective and approach to these highly complex cases.

Preoperative Assessment, Patient Education, and Psychological Preparation

Anesthesia consultation should be scheduled for all patients with placenta accreta prior to the day of surgery. At that point, the anesthesiologist has an opportunity to review the medical records, meet with the patient, and discuss important medical, obstetrical, and anesthetic histories. Additionally, it is equally important to talk with the patient in a detailed, personal, and supportive way about her knowledge of and concerns regarding the upcoming procedure. Level of education, medical knowledge, and worldview may differ substantially among patients. Gaining an understanding about the patient's beliefs, expectations, fears, and preferences allows the anesthesiologist to provide optimal support and improves the patient's experience. The anesthesiologist should manage patient expectations for how the day of surgery will progress, address any concerns, and answer all questions the patient might have. An unhurried and empathetic preoperative meeting between the patient and anesthesiologist helps streamline care and minimize patient anxiety in preparation for surgery.

Medical History

When obtaining a medical history there is particular focus on cardiopulmonary disease, exercise tolerance, spine abnormalities, neurologic deficits or disorders, bleeding and transfusion history, and obstetrical history. Obstetrical patients are often relatively healthy, but with the rise in obesity,[3,4] an aging maternal population,[5,6] and improved management of congenital defects and disorders (i.e., congenital heart defects[7]), obstetrical anesthesiologists encounter an increasingly complex population.

In patients with placenta accreta, who may undergo extensive tissue dissection and are at risk for massive hemorrhage, it is important to take a thorough bleeding history, which is the cornerstone of a hemostatic evaluation.[8] Laboratory tests are not a substitute for a thorough history. Patients should be asked about bleeding in many different ways: Have they ever had surgery or a deep cut? Did they bleed excessively? Have they had their tonsils or adenoids removed? Have they had any dental extractions? Removal of tonsils, adenoids, and teeth constitute potent hemostatic challenges, and a negative history of excessive bleeding after such surgery is important. Patients should also be asked about excessive menstrual bleeding and easy bruising.[9–12] Some degree of gum bleeding or epistaxis can be a normal occurrence in pregnancy.

Assessing bleeding risk and initiating early modification can improve outcomes in patients who are at risk for peripartum hemorrhage.[13] If iron deficiency anemia is identified, iron replacement therapy may be started. Erythropoietin, more often used in anemia associated with renal failure, has been used in pregnancy to increase red blood cell mass.[14–16] Inherited coagulopathies may be managed proactively by having factor replacement therapy available on the day of surgery. Iatrogenic coagulopathies from anticoagulation medication should be documented and managed proactively.

Anticoagulant type, timing, and dose affect feasibility of regional anesthesia.[17–21] Table 11.1 provides a summary of commonly used anticoagulants in pregnancy and implications for placement of neuraxial anesthesia. Active reversal of anticoagulant medication is also managed differently, which is relevant in

TABLE 11.1

Anticoagulation Guidelines for Neuraxial Procedures to Minimize Risk of Hematoma

Medication	Half-Life (hours)	Minimum Time between Last Dose of Anticoagulant and Neuraxial Procedure	With Catheter in Place	Minimum Time between Last Dose of Anticoagulant and Catheter Removal	When to Restart Anticoagulant after Neuraxial Procedure or Catheter Removal
Aspirin[a]	6				
NSAIDs[a]	2–20	May be given, no time restrictions when used alone			
Heparin[b]					
5000 units SC BID	1–2	No contraindication. Per ASRA, consider 8–10 hours hold	Indwelling catheter OK	2–4 hours, ideally remove catheter 1 hour prior to next dose	2 hours

(Continued)

TABLE 11.1 (*Continued*)

Anticoagulation Guidelines for Neuraxial Procedures to Minimize Risk of Hematoma

Medication	Half-Life (hours)	Minimum Time between Last Dose of Anticoagulant and Neuraxial Procedure	With Catheter in Place	Minimum Time between Last Dose of Anticoagulant and Catheter Removal	When to Restart Anticoagulant after Neuraxial Procedure or Catheter Removal
5000 units SC TID		When aPTT<40, 8–10 hours	CONTRAINDICATED		
SC full-dose >10,000 units/day		When aPTT<40, 8–10 hours			
Full-dose IV		When aPTT<40, check after holding 4 hours	CONTRAINDICATED (can give single low-dose IV heparin 2 hours postneuraxial procedure)		
Low-molecular-weight heparin					
Enoxaparin 40 mg SC daily prophylaxis		12 hours	Indwelling catheter OK, can start 4 hours postneuraxial procedure	12 hours	
Enoxaparin 30 mg SC BID prophylaxis		12–24 hours	CONTRAINDICATED	24 hours	
Enoxaparin 1 mg/kg SC BID or 1.5 mg/kg SC daily treatment	4–7	24 hours	CONTRAINDICATED		4 hours
Dalteparin 5000 units SC daily		12 hours	Indwelling catheter OK, can start 4 hours postneuraxial procedure	12 hours	
Dalteparin 200 units/kg SC daily or 120 units/kg SC q12 hours		24 hours	CONTRAINDICATED		

Sources: Narouze S et al., *Reg Anesth Pain Med*, 40, 182–212, 2015; Horlocker TT et al., *Reg Anesth Pain Med*, 35, 35, 64–101, 2010; Gupta R, *APSF*, 2012; Greaves JD, *Anaesthesia*, 52, 150–154, 1997; Sandhu H et al., *Reg Anesth Pain Med*, 25, 72–75, 2000; Cushman M et al., Presented by the American Society of Hematology, adapted in part from the American College of Chest Physicians Evidence-Based Clinical Practice Guideline on Antithrombotic and Thrombolytic Therapy, 2011.

Notes: Assessment of patient risk factors for thrombosis versus bleeding should be made in all cases. Longer hold periods may be considered for patients with impaired renal function or in patients who have a high risk of bleeding and low risk for thrombosis. The presence of blood during the procedure, concomitant aspirin/NSAID use, and heparinization within 1 hour were identified as risk factors for the development of a spinal hematoma.

Abbreviations: NSAIDs, nonsteroidal anti-inflammatory drugs; SC, subcutaneous; BID, "bis in die"—twice a day; ASRA, American Society of Regional Anesthesia; TID, "ter in die"—three times a day; aPTT, activated partial thromboplastin time; IV, intravenous; mg, milligram; kg, kilogram.

a Aspirin/NSAIDs in combination therapy with unfractionated heparin or low-molecular-weight heparin, oral anticoagulants, herbal medications (garlic, ginkgo, willow), and thrombolytics has been shown to increase the frequency of spontaneous hemorrhage.

b Patients taking heparin for >4 days need a platelet count assessed before neuraxial block and catheter removal.

the setting of emergent bleeding. For example, protamine sulfate provides full reversal of unfractionated heparin and only 60%–80% of low-molecular-weight heparin. Protamine dose for reversal of heparin is 1 mg/100 units of heparin given in the previous 2–3 hours, but it is 1 mg of protamine/1 mg of enoxaparin given in the previous 8 hours.[22] There are numerous anticoagulants currently available, all of which have different practice parameters, and discussion of which is beyond the scope of this chapter.

When addressing the issue of bleeding, it is important to identify a patient's willingness to accept blood replacement therapy. Personal belief systems vary, and patients who are unwilling to accept blood products should be identified, counseled, and properly consented prior to the day of surgery. In some cases, patients unwilling to accept allogeneic blood products are willing to accept cell salvage or acute normovolemic hemodilution (ANH), which should be made available.

Cell salvage has been used since the 1970s in nonobstetric hemorrhage as a way to decrease use of allogeneic blood products. Concern for amniotic fluid embolus (AFE) and maternal alloimmunization limited its extension into obstetrics in the past, but it is currently an accepted practice. Red cell washing and leukocyte-reducing filters should eliminate the risk of amniotic fluid contamination. Notably, amniotic fluid contamination of the maternal circulation is similar in cesarean sections with or without the use of cell salvage.[23–27]

ANH is a blood conservation technique that involves removal of blood from the patient prior to surgical incision, with continuous fetal heart rate monitoring in place, and replacement of intravascular volume with colloid or crystalloid to maintain normovolemia. The amount of blood removed varies based on starting maternal hemoglobin and maternal and fetal tolerance of the resulting dilutional anemia. The blood is given back to the patient during or shortly after surgery. ANH is seldom used in obstetrics, but has a role for patients who will not receive allogeneic blood (e.g., Jehovah's Witness) and are expected to hemorrhage.[28]

A witnessed consent of what blood replacement therapies the patient will and will not accept is essential. This is not only important from the patient's perspective but also for care providers involved in the case. Anesthesiologist or surgeons unwilling to forego possible live-saving transfusion interventions should remove themselves from the case and assist the family in finding alternative providers. Hospital ethics committees and risk management are often helpful and may be consulted.

Surgical History

Surgical history, including prior cesarean sections and other abdominal surgeries, add complexity to an already challenging case and may affect the choice of anesthetic. Previous back surgery or scoliosis may affect feasibility and efficacy of regional anesthesia, making general anesthesia a more appropriate choice.[29,30] Anesthetic history including types of anesthetics the patient has had in the past, any adverse reactions such as postoperative nausea and vomiting, history of difficult airway, and personal or family history of malignant hyperthermia will further influence the anesthesiologist's decision-making. If available, a review of prior anesthesia records helps identify and avoid previous problems.

Physical Examination

Physical examination should include, but is not limited to, an airway, heart, and lung examination. Knowledge of and respect for the anatomic and physiologic changes in the obstetrical airway are essential. Increased use of regional anesthesia has arguably led to a lack of familiarity with these changes.[31] Estrogen effects and increased blood volume contribute to edema and vascular congestion of the respiratory tract mucosa, which can lead to mucosal bleeding and difficult endotracheal tube passage. Functional residual capacity (FRC) is the volume of gas remaining in the lung at the end of normal exhalation that serves as a reservoir of oxygen during periods of apnea. Due to the cephalad displacement of the diaphragm by the gravid uterus, FRC is decreased by 20% in the sitting position and up to 25% in the supine position. This decrease in FRC, coupled with increased oxygen consumption and carbon dioxide production during pregnancy speed up the onset of arterial oxygen desaturation during periods of hypoventilation and apnea.[31–33]

An anticipated difficult airway is important to plan for and often leads the anesthesiologist to start the case with a general anesthetic. Emergently securing a difficult airway in the setting of patient discomfort, suboptimal surgical conditions, hemodynamic instability, and/or altered patient consciousness should be avoided. The American Society of Anesthesiologists (ASA) Practice Guidelines for management of difficult airway is a useful resource for airway management.[34]

Assessment of the ease of intravascular (IV) access should be made since multiple peripheral IV lines will need to be placed. The neck should be examined for ease of internal jugular vein access. Notably, central venous catheter (CVC) placement may be more challenging in the obstetrical population and is prone to complications.[35,36] If a CVC is placed, it should be a large-bore sheath introducer, commonly 8 or 9 French diameter, intended for rapid infusion. A rapid infuser catheter (RIC) line provides an excellent alternative to a CVC because it is relatively simple to place, has a 7 or 8.5 French diameter, and is peripherally inserted to minimize the risks otherwise associated with CVCs.

When a regional anesthetic is planned, the back should be examined. Ultrasound-guided spine examination has become more popular in recent years to evaluate and facilitate access to the neuraxial space, especially in patients with obesity, abnormal spine anatomy, or prior back surgery.[37]

Preoperative laboratory assessment should include a basic metabolic panel, complete blood count and type, and crossmatch. The starting hemoglobin and extent of the abnormal placentation often dictate the number of units of blood immediately available on the day of surgery. A massive obstetrical hemorrhage protocol should be in place to facilitate rapid access to blood products.[38,39] A minimum of four units of packed red blood cells (PRBC) and four units of fresh frozen plasma (FFP) should be available prior to surgery and the blood bank must be notified of the severity of the case. Platelets and cryoprecipitate should be prepared in advance on a case-by-case basis if massive hemorrhage is anticipated.

Other laboratory tests should be ordered as indicated by the patient's medical history and current clinical status. For example, a coagulation panel in the setting of recent anticoagulation or electrocardiogram and/or echocardiogram in the setting of cardiovascular disease are indicated.

Intraoperative Management

Ideally, one anesthesia team should provide care for the entirety of the case. In some institutions, patients may be admitted the night before for laboratory assessment and IV placement in preparation for early morning surgery or transport to interventional radiology (IR). If a regional anesthetic is planned, it should be placed and tested by the anesthesiologist assigned to the case before femoral arterial sheaths are in place if IR is to be performed. Institutional practice may vary as to whether the anesthesiologist needs to monitor the patient in IR, but if the patient has not received sedation and the regional block has not been activated this is often unnecessary. Nevertheless, the anesthesiologist, surgical team, and an operating room should remain available while the patient is in IR in case of maternal or fetal decompensation requiring urgent delivery.

Preoperative administration of histamine-2-receptor antagonists and nonparticulate antacids (i.e., sodium citrate or sodium bicarbonate) to reduce gastric acidity is standard practice. Some clinicians may add an antidopaminergic promotility agent such as metoclopromide to reduce the volume of gastric contents. Metoclopromide and H2-receptor antagonists should ideally be given 30 minutes prior to surgery. Nonparticulate antacids should be given within 20 minutes of induction of anesthesia. Pregnant patients are always considered to have a full stomach, but standard nil per os (NPO, nothing by mouth) guidelines of 8 hours from last full meal and 2 hours from last clear liquid intake are maintained for elective surgeries.[40]

Upon arrival to the operating room the patient is transferred to the operating room table and placed in the supine left uterine displacement position to minimize aortocaval compression and optimize maternal-fetal blood flow. Standard ASA monitors will be applied in every case including blood pressure, pulse oximetry, electrocardiogram, end-tidal carbon dioxide, and temperature. Additionally, two large-bore peripheral IV lines and an arterial line are placed, if not already present.

The arterial line allows for continuous blood pressure monitoring and frequent laboratory draws, which become indispensable in cases with large blood loss and fluid shifts requiring massive resuscitation. Hypocalcemia, common in the setting of massive transfusion, is associated with coagulopathies, decreased systemic vascular resistance, and arrhythmias. Metabolic acidosis due to poor organ perfusion is associated with myocardial depression, vasodilation, arrhythmias, decreased thrombin generation, and impaired coagulation.[41] Goal-directed transfusion medicine directed by laboratory results may improve outcomes and reduce blood product administration.[42-45] Having an arterial line makes it easy to trend laboratory results such as calcium, pH, hemoglobin, platelets, coagulation panel, fibrinogen, and the thromboelastogram.

All intravenous fluids should be infused through fluid warmers. Hypothermia leads to decreased synthesis of acute phase proteins and clotting factors, slowing of the coagulation cascade, prolonged clotting time, and decreased citrate metabolism. Every 1°C drop leads to a 10% reduction in coagulation factor activity.[41,46,47] Other consequences of hypothermia include arrhythmias, poor wound healing, increased wound infections, postoperative shivering, and delayed emergence from anesthesia.[48] Therefore, maintenance of normothermia is very important.

Rapid fluid or blood administration can be made with hand-squeezed fluid chambers, pressure bags, or automatic infusion devices, depending on the availability at each individual institution. If pressurized infusion systems are used it is of key importance to eliminate air from all systems, since morbidity and mortality from iatrogenic air embolism have occurred.[49]

Easy access to internal iliac artery balloons, if placed and clearly identified staff responsible for inflating the balloons if/when necessary should be determined during the surgical time out.

Anesthetic Technique

The choice of anesthetic technique is made on an individual basis determined by the anesthesiologist's judgment with special consideration for maternal, fetal, and obstetrical factors. As previously mentioned, there are advantages and disadvantages to each anesthetic option. Regional techniques are preferred to general anesthesia for most cesarean deliveries in current practice,[40] but cases of placenta accreta present unique challenges that may preclude these techniques. Cases expected to have significant intraoperative bleeding and/or placental invasion of the urinary bladder and other pelvic structures are often better managed with general anesthesia.[50]

Regional anesthesia for cesarean section has been associated with a 17-fold decrease in overall complications, including failed intubation, aspiration, hypoxia, intraoperative recall, and maternal death.[51] Additional benefits of regional anesthesia include decreased fetal drug exposure and parental involvement in the delivery. Absolute contraindications for regional anesthesia include patient refusal or inability to cooperate, increased intracranial pressure, skin or soft tissue infection at the site of needle placement, coagulopathy, uncorrected hypovolemia, and inadequate training of the practitioner.[52] An additional consideration for these cases includes the timing of regional anesthesia initiation relative to placement of internal iliac artery balloons. Once groin sheaths are in place, the patient is not able to flex at the hip, which limits positioning. Ideally, placement and assessment of regional anesthesia occur prior to IR balloon placement.

Pain pathways engaged during a cesarean delivery enter the spinal cord from T4 to S4 engaging both visceral and somatic nerve fibers, which must be covered by the regional technique chosen. Due to duration of surgery and desire for hemodynamic stability, practitioners are less likely to use a single shot spinal technique and more commonly use either an epidural or a combined spinal-epidural (CSE). The regional block is activated by local anesthetic. Most practitioners supplement local anesthetic with a short-acting, lipid-soluble opioid such as fentanyl for intraoperative pain control, and long-acting, water-soluble morphine for postoperative pain control.

Spinal anesthesia is achieved by injecting medication into the intrathecal (IT) space after visualization of cerebral spinal fluid (CSF) confirms proper needle location. The use of a small-gauge, pencil point spinal needle decreases the incidence of postdural puncture headache. Doses and drugs used may vary by institution. The block is rapid in onset, dense in quality, and time limited.

Epidural anesthesia is established by accessing the epidural space through a loss of resistance technique, passing a catheter into the epidural space, and dosing the catheter with local anesthetic to achieve an appropriate anesthetic level. Epidural opioids are also given for both intraoperative (fentanyl 50–100 µg) and postoperative (morphine 2–4 mg) pain control. When compared with a spinal anesthetic, epidural placement is technically more difficult, and the block is slower in onset and may be patchier or less dense. Benefits of an epidural over a spinal include unlimited duration of action, gradual onset, and ability to titrate, which offers greater hemodynamic stability.

For a CSE, the epidural space is accessed as above. Then, a spinal needle is placed through the epidural needle to puncture the dura and arachnoid membranes to administer IT medications. The spinal needle is then withdrawn, and a catheter is placed through the epidural needle into the epidural space. The CSE offers the benefits of both a spinal (fast, dense block) and an epidural (extended duration of action). Some practitioners administer opioids only into the IT space and then activate the epidural with local anesthetic, which allows for greater hemodynamic stability and adequate evaluation of the epidural prior to surgical incision.

Continuous spinal anesthesia (CSA) is performed by accessing the IT space with a larger gauge needle, passing a catheter directly into the cerebrospinal fluid, and then administering medication. The block has the benefit of a spinal (fast, bilateral, and dense), but it is more titratable, and the duration can be extended because of the presence of a catheter. The risk of postdural puncture headache is significantly greater with this technique.[53] Additionally, if the IT catheter is mistaken for an epidural catheter, the patient is at risk for a high or total spinal resulting in hypotension, loss of consciousness, respiratory arrest, and even death if unrecognized.

Neuraxial blocks with local anesthetics inhibit sympathetic as well as sensory and motor nerves. This sympathectomy causes vasodilation of both resistance arterioles, which reduces systemic vascular resistance, and venous capacitance vessels, which in turn reduces venous return and cardiac output. In the setting of heavy blood loss, the presence of an irreversible sympathectomy can make resuscitation of the patient more difficult than if a sympathectomy is not present as with general anesthesia. This is a fundamental hemodynamic reason for avoiding neuraxial anesthesia in patients who are expected to have considerable hemorrhage. In addition to hemodynamic instability, concern for coagulation abnormalities, which follow massive resuscitation and increase the risk for epidural hematoma formation, makes general anesthesia a more favorable option.[54]

For general anesthesia, the patient is positioned, adequate preoxygenation is performed, monitors and Foley catheter are placed, prophylactic antibiotics are given, the abdomen is surgically prepped and draped, and surgeons are scrubbed prior to induction. The goal is to minimize anesthetic exposure to the fetus because induction and maintenance agents cross the placenta and can lead to neonatal depression. This plan should be explicitly stated to both the patient and the surgical team to avoid both patient anxiety and a premature skin incision on a patient who is not yet anesthetized.

To facilitate endotracheal intubation, the patient is placed in the "sniffing position" where the external auditory meatus and sternal notch are aligned in the same horizontal plane leading to internal alignment of the oral, pharyngeal, and tracheal axes. Due to the fact that all parturients are considered to have a full stomach, a rapid sequence intubation with cricoid pressure is performed. In the case of a difficult airway, a fiberoptic intubation while the patient is awake may be necessary. Safely securing the maternal airway takes precedence over fetal drug exposure, and intubating under surgical drapes adds complexity to the procedure. Therefore, in the case of anticipated difficult airway, the patient may not be prepped and draped so the anesthesiologist has full, unobstructed access to the patient. Surgeons may make an incision once proper placement of the endotracheal tube is confirmed with bilateral breath sounds and measured end-tidal carbon dioxide.

There are many anesthetic agents for induction and maintenance. A summary of common agents is presented in Table 11.2. Special considerations for the management of a cesarean hysterectomy under general anesthesia include the normal physiologic changes in pregnancy, hemodynamic stability during potentially catastrophic hemorrhage, and fetal/neonatal effects (Table 11.3). Anesthetic requirements for volatile agents are reduced by 25%–40% in pregnancy due to hormonal influences. Additionally, higher levels of volatile agents decrease uterine tone.[56,57] All induction and maintenance drugs for general

TABLE 11.2

Common General Anesthetic Agents Used for Cesarean Hysterectomy

Drug	Dose	Hemodynamics	Comments
Induction Agents			
Propofol	1–2.5 mg/kg (induction), 50–200 mcg/kg/min (maintenance)	↓ CO and MAP; stable HR	Rapid onset hypnotic with no analgesic properties, short duration of action, antiemetic, pain on injection
Etomidate	0.2–0.5 mg/kg	Stable CO, MAP, and HR	Adrenocortical suppression, myoclonus, pain on injection
Ketamine	1–2 mg/kg (induction), 2–15 mcg/kg/min (sedation)	↑ CO, MAP, HR	Bronchodilator, minimal respiratory depression, analgesic properties, hallucinations
Thiopental	4 mg/kg	↓ CO and MAP; myocardial depressant	Rapid onset, bronchospasm with light anesthesia
Maintenance Agents			
Nitrous oxide	MAC 105%	Stable CO, MAP, and HR	No effect on uterine tone, case report of internal iliac artery balloon rupture with N$_2$O use,[55] postoperative nausea
Volatile agents		Varies slightly by agent; ↓ SVR and MAP	Decreased uterine tone, trigger for malignant hyperthermia
Other			
Opioids		↓ HR (except meperidine), relatively stable HD	Analgesia, histamine release with some agents, respiratory depression
Benzodiazepines		Minimal ↓ CO, MAP	Antegrade amnesia, anxiolytic

Source: Kuczkowski KM and Eisenmann UB, *Ann Fran Anesth Reanim*, 24, 564–565, 2005.

Abbreviations: CO, cardiac output; MAP, mean arterial pressure; HR, heart rate; MAC, minimum alveolar concentration—concentration of vapor in lungs needed to prevent movement in 50% of subjects exposed to surgical pain; SVR, systemic vascular resistance.

anesthesia cross the placenta to varying degrees leading to neonatal sedation. Muscle relaxants used for maternal intubation do not cross the placenta. The pediatric or neonatal team should be immediately available in the operating room during delivery.

General anesthesia is more frequently performed for placenta accreta cases. Concerns for hemodynamic instability, risk of coagulopathy, and inability to quickly titrate the level of anesthesia are some of the factors contributing to this preference. Additionally, the surgical incision may need to extend well above the umbilicus, making appropriate anesthetic coverage by a regional block challenging. Some practitioners may elect to start the case under regional anesthesia and convert to general anesthesia after delivery of the baby. The benefits of this approach are that the mother gets to experience the birth of her child, a support person is able to be with the mother during the delivery, there is decreased fetal drug exposure, and postoperative pain control may be offered by regional anesthesia followed by the induction of general anesthesia for the hysterectomy portion of the surgery. Chestnut et al.[58,59] reported that 22%–28% of regional anesthetics were converted to general anesthesia due to inadequate operating conditions and/or patient discomfort during planned cesarean hysterectomies. Therefore, many practitioners prefer general anesthesia from the start of the case to avoid administration of two different anesthetics and having induction of general anesthesia coincide with massive hemorrhage and initiation of resuscitation efforts.[60–70]

TABLE 11.3

Comparison of Anesthetic Options for Cesarean Hysterectomy

	Spinal	Epidural	Combined Spinal Epidural	Continuous Spinal Anesthesia	General Anesthesia
Onset	Fast	Slow	Fast	Fast	Fast
Duration	Time limited	Unlimited	Unlimited	Unlimited	Unlimited
Laterality	No	Possible	Possible with epidural component	No	No
Dural puncture	Yes	No	Yes	Yes, large, significantly higher incidence of PDPH	No
Hemodynamic stability, titratable	Less HD stability, unable to titrate or re-dose	More HD stability, easily titrated	May use lower IT doses to improve HD stability, able to titrate epidural	More HD stability, easily titrated	More HD stability, easily titrated
Postoperative pain control	Yes, IT morphine	Yes, epidural morphine OR continued postoperative infusion with LA ± opioid	Yes, neuraxial morphine OR continued postoperative infusion with LA ± opioid	Yes, IT morphine OR continued postoperative infusion with LA ± opioid	No
Fetal drug exposure	Minimal	Minimal; slightly increased from spinal given larger required drug doses	Minimal	Minimal	Highest; all induction and maintenance drugs cross the placenta
Other	Mother awake; not suitable for long cases and/or cases with large expected blood loss	Mother awake	Mother awake; may not be able to fully assess epidural function	Mother awake; caution with dosing, high, or total spinal can occur if mistaken for epidural	Secured airway in the case of HD instability and uncontrolled hemorrhage; no sympathectomy (unlike regional anesthesia); caution with maternal history of MH or GETA intolerance, difficult airway

Abbreviations: PDPH, postdural puncture headache; HD, hemodynamic; IT, intrathecal; LA, local anesthetic; MH, malignant hyperthermia; GETA, general endotracheal anesthesia.

Postoperative Management and Care

Postoperative recovery location and level of care should be decided prior to surgery so that appropriate nursing staff and bed availability are provided. Patients who are extubated and hemodynamically stable may be able to recover in the postanesthesia care unit. Patients who remain intubated or require continuing hemodynamic support should be transferred directly to a surgical intensive care unit.

Surveillance for and management of postpartum hemorrhage are important. Serial examinations and close monitoring in the postoperative period allow for rapid intervention if necessary. It is our practice to keep one femoral arterial sheath in place postoperatively in the event that the patient requires further IR intervention. Vascular access can be difficult to obtain in a hemorrhaging, unstable patient.

There are many options for pain management after cesarean hysterectomy including neuraxial opioids and local anesthetics, patient controlled analgesia (PCA) pump, intravenous (IV) and/or oral (PO) medication, transverse abdominis plane (TAP) peripheral nerve blocks, and local wound infiltration. Neuraxial morphine provides optimal analgesia peaking at 60–90 minutes and lasting up to 24 hours. Side effects of neuraxial morphine include pruritus, nausea, vomiting, urinary retention, and delayed respiratory depression. Patients require hourly respiratory evaluations for the first 12 hours and then every 2 hours for the next 12 hours after administration of neuraxial morphine. Epidural, CSE, or CSA analgesia with opioids, and/or local anesthetic may be continued in the postoperative period. This is especially useful in patients with a history of chronic pain or chronic opioid use. With IV or PO medications, a multimodal approach is best,[56] including opioids, nonsteroidal anti-inflammatory drugs (NSAIDs), and acetaminophen. NSAIDs such as ibuprofen and ketorolac are useful analgesics, but caution should be used in the setting of renal insufficiency and use may be limited in placenta accreta cases due to concern for platelet dysfunction and suboptimal hemostasis.

Since general anesthesia without regional block placement is more common for the management of placenta accreta, many patients will not receive neuraxial morphine. In such cases, peripheral nerve blocks or local wound infiltration may be considered for postoperative pain management. A TAP block involves injecting local anesthetic into the plane between the internal oblique and transversus abdominis muscles with the intention of blocking innervation to the abdominal skin, muscles, and parietal peritoneum. From a single posterior injection one can expect analgesia from T10 to L1. Of note, the lateral abdominal wall is more densely blocked than the midline, making analgesic coverage better for Pfannenstiel incisions than for midline, vertical incisions. TAP blocks remain inferior to neuraxial morphine for postoperative pain control for cesarean section.[71–73]

Lactation and Nursing

Given the short-and long-term positive effects for both mother and infant, the World Health Organization and the American Academy of Pediatrics recommend exclusive breastfeeding of infants up to 6 months of age followed by continued human milk consumption with introduction of complementary foods for 1 year or more as desired by the mother and infant.[74–76] Since anesthetic agents and analgesic medication are secreted in breast milk, there are theoretical concerns regarding neonatal exposure. One option is to consider pumping and discarding breast milk after exposure and prior to initiation of breastfeeding.

Regional anesthesia often uses a combination of local anesthetic and opioid medications. Local anesthetics are large molecules that do not easily cross into the lactating ducts and transfer into breast milk is minimal. Therefore, neuraxial local anesthetics are safe in breastfeeding mothers. Serum concentration after neuraxially administered opioids depends on the drug, route, dose, and frequency, but levels are often low even if detectable and are considered safe.[74,77]

For general anesthesia, as a practical guideline, once the mother has recovered sufficiently, she may resume breastfeeding, and there is no need to discard her breast milk. Inhalational agents are rapidly excreted and have poor oral bioavailability, making them safe to use in lactating women. Induction agents, such as propofol and etomidate, either have poor infant absorption or drug levels in the breast milk or are so small that breastfeeding may be resumed once the mother has recovered. Oral or IV opioids in multiple-doses or for the management of chronic pain should be used with greater caution and may require further neonatal monitoring as compared with single-doses (fentanyl or morphine), which have minimal neonatal effects. In terms of benzodiazepines, midazolam has a more favorable profile with respect to use in lactating women for premedication or intraoperatively when compared with diazepam and lorazepam. NSAIDs such as ketorolac and ibuprofen may be safely used and have the benefit of being opioid-sparing.[74–83] Specifics regarding different agents and their safety in lactation may be reviewed on the LactMed website at http://toxnet.nlm.nih.gov/cgi-bin/sis/htmlgen?LACT.

Mothers who received general anesthesia in the peripartum or postpartum period have delayed onset of lactation and decreased milk production. Providers should consider avoidance of prolonged fasting times when appropriate and good IV hydration to assist in the production of milk.

Summary

Open, frequent communication and meticulous coordination with the patient, the patient's support system, and various specialists involved are paramount to success. Early diagnosis allows for advanced preparation to take place including referral to a specialty center, hemorrhage risk assessment and modification, multidisciplinary consultation and care conferences, and blood bank notification. Anesthesia consultation prior to the day of surgery is indispensable. The choice of anesthetic is made on case-by-case basis. Factors that play into the decision between a general and regional anesthetic include patient characteristics, extent of placental invasion, surgical technique, and practitioner preference. General anesthesia remains the favored approach for patients with significant risk of massive hemorrhage, profound hypotension, coagulopathy, and extensive surgical manipulation and tissue dissection. Well-functioning institutional protocols for massive hemorrhage must be in place to ensure rapid, efficient, and effective availability and administration of blood products. Additionally, cell salvage is an accepted and valuable resource for obstetrical hemorrhage. Table 11.4 provides a summary of anesthetic considerations for placenta accreta.

TABLE 11.4

Summary of Anesthetic Considerations for Placenta Accreta

Early diagnosis
    Referral to an experienced center with adequate resources and coverage
    Risk assessment: extent of placental invasion, maternal anemia, known coagulopathies, willingness to accept blood replacement therapy
    Risk modification: iron supplementation, availability of replacement factors
    Comprehensive advanced planning
Anesthesia consultation
    Complete history and physical exam
    Management of patient expectations and psychological preparation
Multidisciplinary clinical care conference
    Communication key to success and improved outcomes
    Written plan of care for both scheduled and emergency cesarean hysterectomy made available to all involved providers
Intraoperative management
    One anesthesia team provides all hands-on care
    General vs. regional anesthesia decision made on case-by-case basis
    Minimum of two large-bore peripheral IV lines (14 or 16G) for resuscitation efforts
    Arterial line for close HD monitoring and frequent lab draws
    Consider CO monitoring: hand-held transthoracic echocardiography, esophageal Doppler, Flo-Trac, etc.
    IV fluids on warmers and ready for rapid infusion and/or blood transfusion
    Established, well-functioning OB hemorrhage protocol; blood bank notification and preparedness
Postoperative management
    Continued monitoring for maternal HD stability and PPH, often initially ICU-level care
    Plans for postoperative pain control
    Breastfeeding support and encouragement once mother has recovered from anesthesia, no need to "pump and dump"

Abbreviations: IV, intravenous; G, gauge; HD, hemodynamic; CO, cardiac output; OB, obstetric; PPH, postpartum hemorrhage; ICU, intensive care unit.

Caring for a patient with placenta accreta is an increasingly common and uniquely challenging situation. Placenta accreta is one of the two leading causes of peripartum hemorrhage, and the most common indication for peripartum hysterectomy.[84] Therefore, having a comprehensive and multidisciplinary approach to managing patients diagnosed with placenta accreta is invaluable.

REFERENCES

1. Eller AG, Bennett MA, Sharshiner M, et al. Maternal morbidity in cases of placenta accreta managed by a multidisciplinary care team compared with standard obstetric care. *Obstet Gynecol.* 2011;117:331–337.
2. Wright JD, Herzog TJ, Shah M, et al. Regionalization of care for obstetric hemorrhage and its effect on maternal mortality. *Obstet Gynecol.* 2010;115:1194–1200. doi:10.1097/AOG.0b013e3181df94e8.
3. Helms E, Coulson CC, Galvin SL. Trends in weight gain during pregnancy: A population study across 16 years in North Carolina. *Am J Obstet Gynecol.* 2006;194:32–34.
4. Weiss JL, Malone FD, Emig D, et al. Obesity, obstetric complications and cesarean delivery rate—A population-based screening study. *Am J Obstet Gynecol.* 2004;190:1091–1097.
5. Walker KF, Bugg GJ, Macpherson M, et al. Randomized trial of labor induction in women 35 years of age or older. *NEJM.* 2016;374:813–822.
6. Joseph KS, Allen AC, Dodds L, Turner LA, Scott H, Liston R. The perinatal effects of delayed childbearing. *Obstet Gynecol.* 2005;105:1410–1418.
7. Khairy P, Ouyang DW, Fernandes SM, Lee-Parritz A, Economy KE, Landzberg MJ. Pregnancy outcomes in women with congenital heart disease. *Circulation.* 2006;113:517–524.
8. Sham RL, Francis CW. Evaluation of mild bleeding disorders and easy bruising. *Blood Rev.* 1994;8:98–104.
9. Dilley A, Drews C, Miller C, et al. Von Willebrand disease and other inherited bleeding disorders in women with diagnosed menorrhagia. *Obstet Gynecol.* 2001;97:630–636.
10. Knol HM, Mulder AB, Bogchelman DH, Kluin-Nelemans HC, van der Zee AG, Meijer K. The prevalence of underlying bleeding disorders in patients with heavy menstrual bleeding with and without gynecologic abnormalities. *Am J Obstet Gynecol.* 2013;209:202.e1–202.e7.
11. Kadir RA, Economides DL, Sabin CA, Owens D, Lee CA. Frequency of inherited bleeding disorders in women with menorrhagia. *Lancet.* 1998;351:485–489.
12. Kouides PA. Evaluation of abnormal bleeding in women. *Curr Hematol Rep.* 2002;9:11–18.
13. Fleischer A, Meirowitz N. Care bundles for management of obstetrical hemorrhage. *Semin Perinatol.* 2016;40:99–108.
14. Wortman AC, Alexander JM. Placenta accreta, increta, and percreta. *Obstet Gynecol Clin N Am.* 2013;40:137–154.
15. Krafft A, Bencaiova G, Breymann C. Selective use of recombinant human erythropoietin in pregnant patients with severe anemia or nonresponsive to iron sucrose alone. *Fetal Diagn Ther.* 2009;25:239–245.
16. Harris SA, Payne G Jr, Putman JM. Erythropoietin treatment of erythropoietin deficient anemia without renal disease during pregnancy. *Obstet Gynecol.* 1996;87:812–814.
17. Narouze S, Benzon HT, Provenzano DA, et al. Interventional spine and pain procedures in patients on antiplatelet and anticoagulant medications: Guidelines from the American Society of Regional Anesthesia and Pain Medicine, the European Society of Regional Anaesthesia and Pain Therapy, the American Academy of Pain Medicine, the International Neuromodulation Society, the North American Neuromodulation Society, and the World Institute of Pain. *Reg Anesth Pain Med.* 2015;40:182–212.
18. Horlocker TT, Wedel DJ, Rowlingson JC, et al. Regional anesthesia in the patient receiving antithrombotic or thrombolytic therapy: American Society of Regional Anesthesia and Pain Medicine Evidence-Based Guidelines (Third Edition). *Reg Anesth Pain Med.* 2010;35:64–101.
19. Gupta, R. New anticoagulants present new challenges. *APSF.* 2012 http://www.apsf.org/newsletters/html/2012/spring/05_anticoagulant.htm.
20. Greaves JD. Serious spinal cord injury due to haematomyelia caused by spinal anaesthesia in a patient treated with low-dose heparin. *Anaesthesia.* 1997;52:150–154.
21. Sandhu H, Morley-Forster P, Spadafora S. Epidural hematoma following epidural analgesia in a patient receiving unfractionated heparin for thromboprophylaxis. *Reg Anesth Pain Med.* 2000;25:72–75.

22. Cushman M, Lim W, Zakai NA. 2011 Clinical Practice Guide on Anticoagulant Dosing and Management of Anticoagulant-Associated Bleeding Complications in Adults, Presented by the American Society of Hematology, adapted in part from the: American College of Chest Physicians Evidence-Based Clinical Practice Guideline on Antithrombotic and Thrombolytic Therapy (8th Edition), 2011.

23. Araki Y, Fukuda I, Kamiya I, Tsujimoto Y, Sugahara S, Kazama T. Case of cesarean section using Cell Saver5+ in a patient with the placenta accreta associated with massive hemorrhage. *Masui.* 2009;58:499–502.

24. Allahdin S, Voight S, Htwe TT. Management of placenta praevia and accreta. *J Obstet Gynaecol.* 2011;31:1–6.

25. Catling SJ, Freites O, Krishnan S, Gibbs R. Clinical experience with cell salvage in obstetrics: four cases from one UK centre. *Int J Obstet Anesth.* 2002;11:128–134.

26. Waters JH, Lukauskiene E, Anderson ME. Amniotic fluid removal during cell salvage in the caesarean section patient. *Anaesthesiology.* 2000;92:1531–1536.

27. Elagamy A, Abdelaziz A, Ellaithy M. The use of cell salvage in women undergoing cesarean hysterectomy for abnormal placentation. *IJOA.* 2013;22:289–293.

28. Nagy CJ, Wheeler AS, Archer TL. Acute normovolemic hemodilution, intra-operative cell salvage and pulseCO hemodynamic monitoring in a Jehovah's Witness with placenta percreta. *Inter J Obstet Anesth.* 2008;17:159–163.

29. Ko JY, Leffert LR. Clinical implications of neuraxial anesthesia in the parturient with scoliosis. *Anesth Analg.* 2009;109:1930–1934.

30. Bauchat JR, McCarthy RJ, Koski TR, Wong CA. Labor analgesia consumption and time to neuraxial catheter placement in women with a history of surgical correction for scoliosis: A case-matched study. *Anesth Analg.* 2015;121:981–987.

31. Mushambi MC, Jaladi S. Airway management and training in obstetric anesthesia. *Curr Opin Anethesiol.* 2016;29. doi:10.1097/ACO.0000000000000309.

32. Kinsella SM, Winton AL, Mushambi MC, et al. Failed tracheal intubation during obstetric general anesthesia: A literature review. *Int J Obstet Anesth.* 2015;24:356–374.

33. Vasdev GM, Harrison BA, Keegan MT, Burkle CM. Management of the difficult and failed airway in obstetric anesthesia. *J Anesth.* 2008;22:38–48.

34. Apfelbaum JL, Hagberg CA, Caplan RA, et al. Practice guidelines for management of the difficult airway: An updated report by the American Society of Anesthesiologists Task Force on Management of the Difficult Airway. *Anesthesiology.* 2013;118:251–270.

35. Nuthalapaty FS, Beck MM, Mabie WC. Complications of central venous catheters during pregnancy and postpartum: A case series. *Obstet Gynecol.* 2009;201:311e1–311e5.

36. Siddiqui N, Goldszmidt E, Haque SU, Carvalho JCA. Ultrasound simulation of internal jugular vein cannulation in pregnant and nonpregnant women. *Can J Anaesth.* 2010;57:966–972.

37. Chin KJ, Perlas A. Ultrasonography of the lumbar spine for neuraxial and lumbar plexus blocks. *Curr Opin Anaesthesiol.* 2011;24:567–572.

38. Butwick AJ, Goodnough LT. Transfusion and coagulation management in major obstetric hemorrhage. *Curr Opin Anaesthesiol.* 2015;28:275–284.

39. Kacmar RM, Mhyre JM, Scavone BM, Fuller AJ, Toledo P. The use of postpartum hemorrhage protocols in United States academic obstetric anesthesia units. *Anesth Analg.* 2014;119:906–910.

40. American Society of Anesthesiologists Task Force of Obstetric Anesthesia. Practice guidelines for obstetric anesthesia: An updated report by the American Society of Anesthesiologists Task Force on Obstetric Anesthesia. *Anesthesiology.* 2016;124. doi:10.1097/ALN.0000000000000935.

41. Sihler KC, Napolitano LM. Complications of massive transfusion. *Chest.* 2010;137:209–220.

42. Yin J, Zhao Z, Li Y, et al. Goal-directed transfusion protocol via thromboelastography in patients with abdominal trauma: A retrospective study. *World J Emerg Surg.* 2014;9:28.

43. Shore-Lesserson L, Manspeizer HE, DePerio M, Francis S, Vela-Cantos F, Ergin MA. Thromboelastography-guided transfusion algorithm reduces transfusions in complex cardiac surgery. *Anesth Analg.* 1999;88:312–319.

44. Afshari A, Wikkelsø A, Brok J, Møller AM, Wetterslev J. Thrombelastography (TEG) or thromboelastometry (ROTEM) to monitor haemotherapy versus usual care in patients with massive transfusion. *Cochrane Database Syst Rev.* 2011 doi:10.1002/14651858.CD007871.pub2.

45. Bolliger D, Gorlinger K, Tanaka KA. Pathophysiology and treatment of coagulopathy in massive hemorrhage and hemodilution. *Anesthesiology.* 2010;113:1205–1219.
46. Watts DD, Trask A, Soeken K, et al. Hypothermic coagulopathy in trauma: Effect of varying levels of hypothermia on enzyme speed, platelet function, and fibrinolytic activity. *J Trauma.* 1998;44:846–854.
47. Wolberg AS, Meng ZH, Monroe III DM, Hoffman MA. Systematic evaluation of the effect of temperature on coagulation enzyme activity and platelet function. *J Trauma.* 2004;56:1221–1228.
48. Kurz A. Thermal care in the perioperative period. *Best Pract Res Clin Anaesthesiol.* 2008;22:39–62.
49. Zoremba N, Gruenewald C, Zoremba M, Rossaint R, Schaelte G. Air elimination capability in rapid infusion systems. *Anaesthesia.* 2011;66:1031–1034.
50. Kuczkowski KM. A review of current anesthetic concerns and concepts for cesarean hysterectomy. *Curr Opin Obstet Gynecol.* 2011;23:401–407.
51. Lynch J, Scholz S. Anaesthetic-related complications of cesarean section. *Zentralbl Gynakol.* 2005;127:91–95.
52. Wong C. Epidural and spinal analgesia/anesthesia for labor and vaginal delivery. In Chestnut DH, ed. *Obstetric Anesthesia: Principles and Practice,* 4th Ed. Philadelphia, PA: Elsevier Mosby; 2009:430.
53. Peyton PJ. Complications of continuous spinal anesthesia. *Anaesth Intensive Care.* 1992;20:417–425.
54. Snegovskikh D, Clebone A, Norwitz E. Anesthetic management of patients with placenta accreta and resuscitation strategies for associated massive hemorrhage. *Curr Opin Anaesthesiol.* 2011;24:274–281.
55. Kuczkowski KM, Eisenmann UB. Nitrous oxide as a cause of internal iliac artery occlusion balloon rupture. *Ann Fran Anesth Reanim.* 2005;24:564–565.
56. Sumikura, H, Niwa H, Sato M, Nakamoto T, Asai T, Hagihira S. Rethinking general anesthesia for cesarean section. *J Anesth.* 2016;30:268–273.
57. Devroe S, Van de Velde M, Rex S. General anesthesia for caesarean section. *Curr Opin Anaesthesiol.* 2015;28:240–246.
58. Chestnut DH, Dewan DM, Redick LF, Caton D, Spielman FJ. Anesthetic management for obstetric hysterectomy: A multi-institutional study. *Anesthesiology.* 1989;70:607–610.
59. Chestnut DH, Redick LF. Continuous epidural anesthesia for elective cesarean hysterectomy. *South Med J.* 1985;78:1168–1169.
60. Ioscovich A, Shatalin D, Butwick AJ, Ginosar Y, Orbach-Zinger S, Weiniger CF. Israeli survey of anesthesia practice related to placenta previa and accreta. *Acta Anaesthesiologica Scandinavica.* 2016;60:457–464. doi:10.1111/aas.12656.
61. Weiniger CF, Einav S, Deutsch L, Ginosar Y, Ezra Y, Eid L. Outcomes of prospectively-collected consecutive cases of antenatal-suspected placenta accreta. *Int J Obstet Anesth.* 2013;22:273–279.
62. Shaylor R, Ginosar Y, Avidan A, Eventov-Friedman S, Amison N, Weiniger CF. Pre-delivery remifentanil infusion for placenta accreta cesarean delivery under general anesthesia: An observational study. *J Matern Fetal Neonatal Med.* 2015;29:2793–2797. doi:10.3109/14767058.2015.1104297.
63. Kuczkowski KM, Miller T. Cesarean hysterectomy for placenta percreta invading the anterior abdominal wall: Anesthetic considerations: A case report. *Middle East J Anesthesiol.* 2008;19:1105–1109.
64. Murata H, Hara T, Sumikawa K. Anesthesia for cesarean hysterectomy in a parturient with placenta accreta. *Masui.* 2009;58:903–906.
65. Kato R, Terui K, Yokota K, Watanabe M, Uokawa R, Miyao H. Anesthetic management for cases of placenta accreta presented for cesarean section: A 7-year single center experience. *Masui.* 2008;57:1421–1426.
66. Eller AG, Porter TF, Soisson P, Silver RM. Optimal management strategies for placenta accreta. *BJOG.* 2009;116:648–654.
67. Russo M, Krenz EI, Hart SR, Kirsch D. Multidisciplinary approach to the management of placenta accreta. *Ochsner J.* 2011;11:84–88.
68. Kuczkowski K. Anesthesia for the repeat cesarean section in the parturient with abnormal placentation: What does an obstetrician need to know? *Arch Gynecol Obstet.* 2006;273:319–321.
69. Gallos G, Redai I, Smiley RM. The role of the anesthesiologist in the management of obstetric hemorrhage. *Semin Perinatol.* 2009;33:116–123.
70. Lilker SJ, Meyer RA, Downey KN, Macarthur AJ. Anesthetic considerations for placenta accreta. *Int J Obstet Anesth.* 2011;20:288–292.

71. Abdallah FW, Halpern SH, Margarido CB. Transversus abdominis plane block for postoperative analgesia after Caesarean delivery performed under spinal anaesthesia: A systematic review and meta-analysis. *Br J Anaesth.* 2012;109:679–687.

72. Eslamian L, Jalili Z, Jamal A, Marsoosi V, Movafegh A. Transversus abdominis plane block reduces postoperative pain intensity and analgesic consumption in elective cesarean delivery under general anesthesia. *J Anesth.* 2012;26:334–338.

73. McDonnell NJ, Paech MJ. The transversus abdominis plane block and post-caesarean analgesia: Are we any closer to defining its role? *Int J Obstet Anesth.* 2012;21:109–111.

74. Dalal PG, Bosak J, Berlin C. Safety of breastfeeding infant after maternal anesthesia. *Pediatr Anesth.* 2013;24:359–371.

75. American Academy of Pediatrics. Policy statement: Breastfeeding and the use of human milk. *Pediatrics.* 2012;129:e827–e841.

76. WHO. World Health Organization Recommendations. Available at: http://www.who.int/topics/breast-feeding/en/. Accessed on January 15, 2017.

77. Cobb B, Liu R, Valentine E, Onuoha O. Breastfeeding after anesthesia: A review for anesthesia providers regarding the transfer of medications into breast milk. *Transl Perioper Pain Med.* 2015;1:1–7.

78. Esener Z, Sarihasan B, Güven H, Ustün E. Thiopentone and etomidate concentrations in maternal and umbilical plasma, and in colostrum. *Br J Anaesth.* 1992;69:586–588.

79. Dailland P, Cockshott ID, Lirzin JD, et al. Intravenous propofol during cesarean section: Placental transfer, concentrations in breast milk, and neonatal effects. A preliminary study. *Anesthesiology.* 1989;71:827–834.

80. Nitsun M, Szokol JW, Saleh HJ, et al. Pharmacokinetics of midazolam, propofol, and fentanyl transfer to human breast milk. *Clin Pharmacol Ther.* 2006;79:549–557.

81. Andersen LW, Qvist T, Hertz J, Mogensen F. Concentrations of thiopentone in mature breast milk and colostrum following an induction dose. *Acta Anaesthesiol Scand.* 1987;31:30–32.

82. Lee JJ, Rubin AP. Breast feeding and anaesthesia. *Anaesthesia.* 1933;48:616–625.

83. Mayo CW, Schlicke CP. Appearance of a barbiturate in human milk. *Proc Staff Meet Mayo Clin.* 1942;17:87–88.

84. Wright JD, Devine P, Shah M, et al. Morbidity and mortality of peripartum hysterectomy. *Obstet Gynecol.* 2010;115:1187–1193.

Index

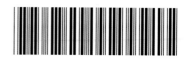